Contents

Introduction	5
How to Use This Book	6
Chapter One: Bringing Out Newborns & Young Infants	13
Chapter Two: Bringing Out Creepers, Crawlers & Toddlers	21
Multiple Locations	23
Central Seattle	32
Indoor Activities	32
Outdoor Activities	39
Montlake, Madison Park, Capitol Hill & Central Area	39
Queen Anne	42
Magnolia	44
North Seattle	47
Indoor Activities	47
Outdoor Activities & Beaches	69
Green Lake, Wallingford & Ravenna	69
Haller Lake, Northgate, Bitter Lake & Lake City	73
Laurelhurst & View Ridge	79
Ballard, Fremont & Phinney Ridge	83
Crown Hill & Loyal Heights	88
Shoreline	90

    Mercer Island, South Seattle and West Seattle 91
        Indoor Activities 91
        Outdoor Activities & Beaches 96
            Mercer Island 96
            Mount Baker, Rainier Valley, & Madrona 98
            West Seattle 102
    The Eastside 108
        Indoor Activities 108
        Outdoor Activities & Beaches 123
            Bellevue & Medina 123
            Kirkland & Redmond 132
            Newcastle, Issaquah & Renton 142

Chapter Three: Bringing Out Baby Shopping
    & Dining 147
        Shopping 147
            Shopping Malls 148
        Restaurants 158

Quick Reference Guide 175
        Top Ten Indoor Locations 175
        Top Ten Outdoor Locations 176
        Program For Early Parent Support (Peps) 177
        Movement Classes 178
        Music Classes 179
        Arts and Crafts 181
        Drop-Off Classes 182
        Dance Classes 182
        Mom with Baby Fitness Classes 183
        Indoor Playgrounds, Open Gyms & Playrooms 184

Index 187

Bringing OUT Baby

SEATTLE & THE EASTSIDE

Places to Take Babies & Toddlers

Julia Rader Detering

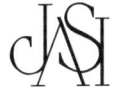

Bringing Out Baby: Seattle & the Eastside–Places to take babies and toddlers
© 1999 by Julia Rader Detering

All rights reserved. This book may not be reproduced in whole or in part by any means without permission from the publisher.

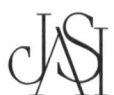
P.O. Box 313
Medina, Washington 98039
(425)454-3490; fax: (425)462-1335
e-mail: jasibooks@aol.com

ISBN 1-881409-50-3
Cover and book design: Marge Mueller, Gray Mouse Graphics
Production, typesetting, and layout: Marge Mueller, Gray Mouse Graphics

Printed in the United States of America

Library of Congress Cataloging-in-Publication Data

Detering, Julia Rader, 1963–
    Bringing out baby : Seattle & the Eastside : places to take babies and toddlers / Julia Rader Detering
      p. cm.
    Includes index.
    ISBN 1-881409-50-3
      1. Seattle Region (Wash.) Guidebooks. 2. Family recreation--Washington (State)--Seattle Region Guidebooks. 3. Mothers--Washington (State) Seattle Region. 4. Infants--Washington (State)--Seattle Region. 5. Toddlers--Washington (State)--Seattle Region. I. Title.
F899.S43D48 1999
917.97'7720443--dc21   99-40753
                                                      CIP

Introduction

My son was born on a rainy night in early December, and it continued to rain and snow for much of the next six weeks. After surviving the first weeks of motherhood, I realized that my baby and I needed to get out of the house.

I joined the support group Program for Early Parent Support (PEPS) and was able to leave my house at least once a week and socialize with other new mothers. By the time I was able to get more sleep and my baby was crying a lot less, I realized I needed more outside contacts.

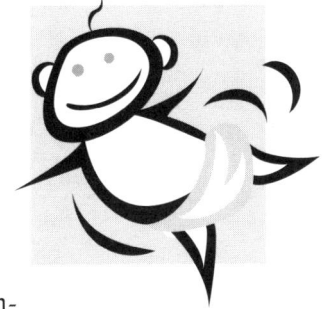

Summertime brought visits to neighborhood parks with the mothers and infants I met in the support group. For the fall I enrolled my baby in a cooperative preschool, a music class and a movement class. Then he got a cold that turned into viral asthma, which landed him in Children's Hospital. His pediatrician advised me to scratch the weekly programs, which would expose him to a multitude of cold and flu viruses, and to become a shut-in for the winter.

Come December, with my baby a year old, I was climbing the walls. I decided to explore Seattle's parks and playgrounds and indoor playgrounds at community centers. I sought out resource guides for more places to take my son, but information was scant. I was disheartened to find that most of the well-publicized activities are for children over three. Thus, the idea for *Bringing Out Baby* was born.

While researching this book, I discovered a plethora of indoor entertainment for even the youngest babies, as well as outside parks and playgrounds that meet a baby's needs for shade, wading pools, or tot swings.

Working parents may feel that they do not have the opportunity to participate in activities that provide bonding experiences with their babies. Fortunately, there are plenty of places that offer activities during evenings and weekends. In each indoor entry I indicate if evening or weekend times are available. Since working mothers usually have at least six weeks of maternity leave, the section titled, Bringing Out Newborns and Young Infants, provides a chance for these mothers to get out with their baby before returning to full-time work.

How to Use this Book

This book you will lead you to a wealth of interesting places and stimulating activities for children under three. Because there is such a broad range of information here, it is difficult to neatly categorize everything. To help you find the place that is perfect for your child, the information has been organized into three chapters.

Chapter One: Newborns & Young Infants

Places where babies can be taken during the first months of their lives are listed in the chapter titled *Bringing Out Newborns & Young Infants*. This chapter provides the names, phone numbers and descriptions of support groups, post-partum exercise programs and infant massage classes. Support groups and exercise programs provide an opportunity for mothers to do something for themselves while still being with their new baby. Any classes, programs or groups listed in chapter one encourage you to bring your baby.

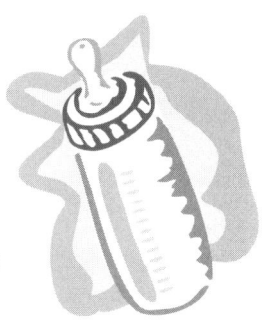

Chapter Two: Creepers, Crawlers & Toddlers

Once babies begin to move about, their interests expand and they are ready for a variety of activities. Chapter two, titled *Bringing Out Creepers, Crawlers & Toddlers* includes those places that are most appropriate for babies whose world has broadened because of their growing mobility and continued developmental advancement.

Because of the wide range of activities babies can enjoy after about six months of age, this chapter includes by far the most information. At the beginning of chapter two is a section titled *Multiple Locations*. This section includes those organizations, both public and private, that offer the same type of program at multiple locations. Libraries with storytime for toddlers, swim classes for infants and Kindermusik classes fall into this category. The activity is described, and then all the locations are listed.

After the Multiple Locations, the creepers, crawlers and toddlers chapter has been divided into four geographic areas. In each of these areas you will find subsections titled *Indoor Sites* and *Outdoor Activities & Beaches*. Indoor sites are listed alphabetically. Because outdoor activities and beaches are so numerous, they are first divided into neighborhoods within each area, then listed alphabetically.

The subsections titled "Indoor Activities" describe community centers in the Seattle area and the Eastside that offer appropriate activities for infants and toddlers, as well as a multitude of nonprofit and private organizations with classes available for children under three.

The subsections titled "Outdoor Activities & Beaches" detail parks and playgrounds that are suitable for youngsters under three years old. To investigate suitable outdoor sites, I visited parks and playgrounds in Seattle, Shoreline, Bellevue, Kirkland, Redmond, Issaquah, and Renton. Parks that offer only playfields, are unkempt or are mostly used by older children are not included in this book. Although I gave some parks and playgrounds a low rating, I felt they were worth mentioning for the benefit of those who live nearby and need a place to stroll. Since a baby that is not yet crawling does not need much of a playground, I included many parks that do not have any play equipment.

Seattle has done a wonderful job of preserving land designated for recreation. Funds have recently been allocated for the upkeep of parks and many playgrounds are being refurbished. Beaches are wonderful places to visit on warm days and abound near the various bodies of water that surround Seattle. Beaches described are those that are especially suitable for babies.

Chapter Three: Shopping & Dining

A third chapter, *Bringing Out Baby Shopping & Dining*, will help you find malls, shopping centers, and restaurants that are child-friendly, and that offer some stimulation for your child. In addition to describing the locations, a few tips are offered for keeping your child happy in restaurants.

Shopping malls provide a great place to get out of the house and stay out of the rain for children of all ages and adults. The major malls in the Seattle area are outlined with the names of baby stores, toy stores and toddler food sources. The location

How to Use this Book

of nursing and diaper changing areas are listed as well.

Restaurants that welcome small children are essential for family. The "kid friendly" restaurants listed in chapter three provide toys or crayons and a children's menu.

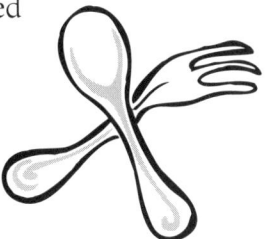

Ratings and Information Blocks

This book's star rating system based on how well the place meets a baby's needs, is intended to help you decide which places may be worth an extra effort to visit. I judged each site by the overall atmosphere, as well as how by much my baby and I enjoyed our visit. The rating levels are:

★★★★ Exceptional
★★★ Very good
★★ OK
★ Not worth any extra effort to visit

In most of the listings, information blocks at the beginning provide a quick summary of what a site has to offer.

Access: Indicates whether there is a parking lot or street parking readily available, and if the site itself can be negotiated with a child in a stroller. Strollers must be able to roll up to the play equipment in order to meet this criterion. For indoor activities, the stroller must be able to roll up to the point of destination.

Hours: For museums, zoos, and centers, the hours of operations are listed.

Fees: For museums and zoos admission fees are listed. Class fees are usually not listed, as they vary and change often. Call the facility for current information about classes offered and fees.

Classes: Indoor entries list classes available for children under three. Since the schedules are constantly changing, it is best to call to inquire about the times and fees of each class.

Weekend/evening hours: This category offers a quick reference for working parents looking for indoor activities that have classes or playrooms available in the evenings or weekends. If no classes are offered on the weekends or evenings it will be noted.

Features: This category lists those things that will be appropriate for your child, and that will make your visit easier.

Parks and playgrounds may have a variety of play equipment. A slide is mentioned if it is suitable for a small child; most tunneled and curved slides are inappropriate. Only swings suitable for tots are listed. Jungle gyms are included in the climber category; unusual climbers are usually described in detail in text. A spinner is the apparatus, also known as a merry-go-round, that a child sits or stands on while a parent spins it. A bouncer is an apparatus shaped like an animal or car, and mounted on a steel coil.

If there is a wading pool, the Wading Pool Hotline number is given; call for times and dates that the pool is open.

In playgrounds, play area surfaces are described. Sand is good for children over a year old, when they can use shovels and pails and no longer eat it or throw it. Gravel and pebbles can be hard for a new walker. Wood chips are the surface of choice in new playgrounds.

Many restrooms at indoor locations have changing tables. Restrooms in parks are often closed for the winter.

Most community centers have vending machines for both food and drink, while many of the private businesses and parks are located near restaurants, cafes, fast-food stops or grocery stores.

A large park with quiet, semiprivate nooks meets the requirement for nursing privacy. Indoor activities that cater to new mothers put a nursing mother at ease, and in these places privacy is not necessary.

Shady spots must be easily available in order to meet this criterion.

When significant features that you may want, such as restrooms, are *not* present they are listed in italic at the end of the information block.

Quick Reference Guide

A quick reference guide at the end of the book provides a list of the top ten indoor and outdoor locations and activities sorted by type, such as movement classes.

* * *

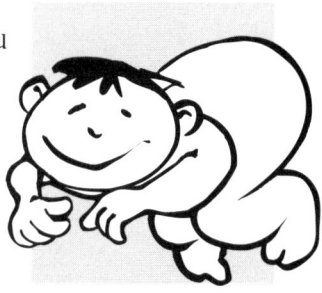

I hope that through this book you will discover activities for your child that you never realized were available. My message to you is this: Get out of the house, and take that precious new life with you. You will both be enriched by the experience.

CHAPTER • ONE

Bringing OUT Newborns & Young Infants

The period when your infant is immobile is precious indeed. Many parents of young children told me to dine out while my infant was very young because later I would not be able take him to restaurants. Now that I have a toddler, I completely understand that advice. Unfortunately, some of us have infants with colic that heats up right around dinner time. For this small but loud group of infants, dining out is simply not an option.

Fortunately, special activities are available that can be done only with infants under four months old. My son was over four months old when I began researching this book, so we could not participate in every activity. I researched them by observing the class or interviewing the instructor or coordinator. In all cases I was able to visit the location of each program to gain a better idea of the parking, restrooms and food availability.

One of the support groups I did participate in was Program for Early Parent Support (PEPS). I had heard about PEPS through friends and was eager to join after I had my child. I strongly recommend this program for every new mother. Even if you are on maternity leave for only a short while, the companionship and comfort you will be afforded is well worth even a brief exposure.

Most of the programs and classes available to mothers of small infants are especially designed for these babies. The exercise classes are called "post-partum" aerobics. Massage classes are designed for babies that lie still. The support groups begin when your baby is a newborn and continue as your baby ages.

Again, I strongly recommend getting out of the house with your young infant. It was very easy to become a shut-in after my son was born. I felt overweight and unattractive, and I was tired all the time. When I started going to PEPS once a week, it forced me to get myself together, thus helping me build back my self-esteem and energy. I hope the research I have done will motivate you to get up and out of the house. Outside activities are a must for both you and your baby.

EVERGREEN COMMUNITY HEALTH CARE   (425)899–3000
12040 NE 128th Street, Kirkland

Hours and fees: Call for class times and fees
Access: Parking available; stroller access
Classes: Parent/Baby Group (0–3 months), (3–6 months), (6–12 months); Young Moms Support Group (0–open age); Yoga for New Moms (up to 6 months)
Features: Restrooms, nursing privacy, changing table, food and drink in cafeteria

    Parent/Baby Group. A group of mothers, fathers or caregivers take their infants to this informal support group. Chairs are placed in a large circle and the babies are put in the middle where they play and socialize while the parents participate in a group discussion. Each week a different topic is discussed. Typically, topics include "The Multi-Dimensional Mom," "Guilt and Motherhood," "Wearing Your Baby" and "Safety for Toddlers." The groups, which meet once a week, are divided by the aforementioned ages. This is a good way to pick up valuable parenting information as well as socialize with other parents.
    Young Moms Support Group. For 1½ hours, new mothers between the ages of fourteen and twenty-two have an opportunity to meet as a group to discuss topics, issues and concerns. A registered nurse facilitates the meetings, but the group helps to decide which issues will be discussed. Mothers take their babies to the class, and bring along their own toys for older babies. The class is free, but mothers must register so they can be notified in case of cancellation or schedule change.
    Yoga for New Moms. Yoga is an excellent way for new mothers to begin the journey back to their pre-pregnancy body. This 1½

hour class is offered in eight-week sessions. Please speak with your health care provider for recommendations on when you can start an exercise program.

Occasionally, Evergreen Hospital also offers Infant Massage. Call the Evergreen Health Line to inquire about other seminars on various topics of interest.

HOLISTIC YOGA CENTER (206)547–9882

4649 Sunnyside Avenue N, Room 300, North Seattle

Hours and fees: Call for class times and fees
Access: Parking available; stroller access
Classes: Post-Natal Yoga (infants); Infant Massage (pre-crawlers)
Features: Restrooms, nursing privacy, food and drink in vending machines

No changing table

Post-Natal Yoga. Whether you have experienced yoga before or if you are a beginner, this form of exercise is a gentle way to get back into shape. The class requires no registration or commitment. Mothers and infants can come only when they feel up to it. The teacher is aware that some mothers have had cesarean sections and require a slower pace. The class is held in the yoga room at the Good Shepherd building. Anywhere from five to twenty-three moms show up at to the classes. Mothers are required to be at least four weeks post-partum, and can bring babies up to a year old as long as the child is quiet enough to allow the mom to participate in the class.

Infant Massage. This class is ideal for babies with colic. The one-hour class is part of a four-class series. Usually five people attend but there is a limit of ten. Lotion and a book are provided.

LA LECHE LEAGUE (206)522–1336–Helpline

Hours and fees: Call for class times and fees
Access: Parking available; stroller access varies
Classes: Meet once a month
Features: Restrooms, changing table availability varies, food and drink availability varies, nursing privacy

La Leche League was founded in 1956 by women who had overcome obstacles associated with breastfeeding. It now serves as a support group and advisor for women who are breastfeeding their babies. The meeting I attended was at the Fremont Baptist Church and was held in the evening. About twenty women with their babies sat in a large circle and exchanged thoughts, concerns and questions about breastfeeding.

The La Leche League leader serves as a facilitator of the meeting and addresses questions asked by the nursing mothers. You do not have to be a mother of a newborn to join the meetings. My baby was four months old when I attended because I was concerned about nursing him to sleep. A friend's child was eighteen months old when she wanted to learn about weaning. There were babies of all ages at the meeting, and all sorts of issues were discussed. The La Leche League leader in your area will also help individually with any nursing problem or concern.

Classes are held all over the Seattle and Greater Seattle area. Call the hotline for class locations and dates.

MOM'S GROUP: SUPPORT GROUP

See page 115.

MOTHERS AND OTHERS: SUPPORT GROUP

See page 116.

Bringing Out Newborns & Young Infants

OVERLAKE HOSPITAL MEDICAL CENTER (425)688-5259

1035 116th Avenue NE, Bellevue

Hours and fees: Call for class times and fees
Access: Parking available; stroller access
Classes: You and Your New Baby (infants 2–12 weeks); Just For Dads (infants 2–12 weeks)
Features: Restrooms, changing table, nursing privacy

No food or drink

You and Your Baby. Between twelve to fifteen mothers with their infants meet for two hours once a week for five weeks in this class. The time is spent learning interesting things about infants. Topics include new parent issues, sick baby dilemmas and infants' nutritional needs.

Just For Dads. Dads take their young infants to this ninety-minute class to learn about the transition from couplehood to parenthood and learn supportive skills for the mother.

Overlake Hospital is planning an infant massage class in the future and also offers a great many courses and lectures for parents in which children do not attend. Call for information.

PROGRAM FOR EARLY PARENT
SUPPORT (PEPS) (206)547-8570

4649 N Sunnyside Avenue, Wallingford

Hours and fees: Call for class times and fees
Classes: Support group meetings
Access: Parking available; stroller access varies
Features: Restrooms, changing table, nursing privacy, snack provided

PEPS provides new parents with support and information in three different programs: Neighborhood, Community, and Teen Parent. The Neighborhood program is available to parents with babies under six months old. In this program, eight to twelve new mothers/fathers and a volunteer facilitator, often a previous PEPS participant, meet for two hours once a week. Generally, everyone lives in the same neighborhood, so the meetings rotate from home to home. During the first hour the leader facilitates a discussion. The second hour is for free talk, singing to the babies, and snacks for the adults. The discussions are informal, but also informative. Often first-time parents have no idea what normal behavior and emotions are for infant, mother, or father. It is helpful to hear how other parents deal with colic, sleeping, and nursing and eventually weaning, feeding, and napping.

Although, I was hesitant to join a group of strangers to discuss something so personal as child-rearing I am glad I participated. Sharing my misery as well as my joy with others helped me through the hard times, and made the good times even more enjoyable.

The Community Program is an excellent alternative to the Neighborhood Program. The free PEPS Parent/Child Activity Time is located at family support centers throughout Seattle. These meetings are available to parents with children under three and are perfect for those with more than one child.

A detailed description of the program is provided within the entry for each family center. See pages 177-178 for a list of where Parent/Child Activity Time is held. Teen Parent groups are held at GED and Work Training sites.

SWEDISH MEDICAL CENTER   (206)386–3606

1120 Cherry Street, first floor aerobics room, First Hill

Hours and fees: Call for class times and fees
Access: Parking garage and meters; stroller access
Classes: Moms and Babies Exercise (pre-crawlers)
Features: Restrooms, nursing privacy, food and drink in vending machines

No changing table

This very low impact aerobics class is designed especially

for post-partum mothers and their infants. Also included in this one-hour class are stretching and abdominal reconditioning. Since the music is mellow and soft the babies are not disturbed. Between eight to ten mothers take their pre-crawling infants to the large mirrored aerobics room. When I was there, most of the babies were nestled in their car seats; however, I did see one baby sitting up on a blanket playing quietly in the corner.

SWEDISH MEDICAL CENTER/BALLARD (206)781–6344
Instructor: (206)789–3857

5300 NW Tallman Avenue, Room ABC, Ballard

Hours and fees: Call for class times and fees
Access: Parking garage and meters; stroller access
Classes: Moms and Babies Exercise (pre-crawlers)
Features: Restrooms, nursing privacy, food and drink in cafeteria

No changing table

This very low impact to non-impact aerobics class is designed especially for post-partum and pre-natal mothers. The room is on the lower floor of the main building at Swedish Hospital. Mothers are encouraged to bring their newborns into the class. Older siblings are welcome in the on-site childcare that is provided free of charge.

Call the instructor for additional classes held elsewhere.

CHAPTER · TWO

Bringing OUT Creepers, Crawlers & Toddlers

Getting out of the house with your baby is especially important as your child becomes more aware of its surroundings. As soon as your baby starts sitting up it is eager to experience new sensations, and exploring new places together can be stimulating for both of you. The feel of soft grass on tiny toes, the smell of flowering trees, and the sight of older children laughing in the sunshine are all experiences waiting at parks and playgrounds around Seattle.

For inclement weather, numerous indoor

activities and places are available. Most indoor activities are ideal for a baby that can walk, although less-mobile infants can be entertained as well. Community centers, family support centers, and private enterprises offer many classes, play areas, and activities for babies of all ages.

At community centers, classes follow a quarterly schedule; call for schedules and fees, as you will need to register before classes begin. Classes at private facilities often follow a quarterly schedule as well. However, some other types of facilities offer ongoing registration. The cost of classes varies widely—at community centers they usually average under $10 per session and can be as little as $3 per session. Activities at commercial locations most often are more expensive. Most indoor activities offer a free preview of the class; call to inquire if such an option is available.

Probably the most popular recreations are the open gyms and indoor playgrounds located at various community centers. They are available to children under five years old. However, these facilities tend to fill up with running toddlers and therefore can be hazardous for smaller infants. Because they are inexpensive, costing between $1 and $2 per child, they are excellent places to take several children. The hours these facilities are open vary widely, and can change from quarter to quarter so you must always check beforehand. Green Lake Community Center and Ballard Community Center have playrooms that are open most of the time. The other community centers often change their hours.

Both indoor and outdoor playgrounds are wonderful places for young crawlers and walkers to burn off energy and meet other youngsters. These are excellent spots to follow the advice of The American Academy of Pediatrics: "The best way for your child to learn how to behave around other people is to be given plenty of trial runs."

Multiple Locations

The following activities have branches throughout King County. Call for specific information.

★★★★
COOPERATIVE PRESCHOOLS

Cooperative preschools provide a popular venue for you and your baby to interact with other parents and babies. Most community colleges offer some type of cooperative preschool in your area. I recommend these for most people, since many of my friends have enjoyed participating in them.

These preschools begin with babies as young as three months old, and can continue with the same group of children until they reach age five. They are called a cooperative because the parents participate by cleaning up, providing a snack, and fund raising. During each two-hour class, early childhood education specialists lead discussions about child rearing, and time is provided for parents and children to socialize. Singing, stories and supervised playtime are a part of the meetings.

As babies grow older, mothers can trade off time, leaving during the class while their child stays with the remaining parents. The cost of these preschools is much less than a daycare center, but can be more expensive than a class at a community center. These cooperatives fill up quickly so contact them to get on a waiting list as soon as you think you might be interested in them.

The following list of phone numbers will help you find a cooperative preschool near you.

Lake Washington Technical College   (425)739–8100
Redmond, Kirkland

Bellevue Community College (425)641–2366
Bellevue, North Bend, Carnation, Issaquah, May Valley, Preston, Mercer Island

Seattle Central Community College (206)587–6938
Queen Anne, Beacon Hill, Madison Park, Capitol Hill, Madrona, Magnolia, Lakewood

South Seattle Community College (206)938–2278
Lincoln Park, Alki, Arbor Heights, High Point, Vashon

Phinney Neighborhood Preschool Cooperative (206)706–2963
North Seattle

North Seattle Community College (206)527–3783
Ballard, Green Lake, Loyal Heights, Fremont, Wallingford

Shoreline Cooperative Preschool (206)362–3257
2545 NE 200th Street, Seattle

North City Parent Cooperative (206)362–4069
2545 NE 200th Street, Seattle

★★★★
GYMBOREE

Gymboree offers developmental play and exercise for babies and toddlers. Classes are divided into age groups focusing on the baby's developmental stage, with the age range in each class increasing as the child grows. An instructor leads parents and babies in using the equipment provided.

At the beginning of the class the teacher explains the focus of the day. For example, the day we went the focus was on the concepts of fast and slow. The teacher advises parents how to use apparatuses such as a large wedge to demonstrate particular concepts to the child. After this, parents spend most of the time playing with their babies, then the group gathers together for activities such as singing, playing on a large colorful parachute, and blowing bubbles.

These classes may be a little pricey, but babies seem to enjoy them. I took my son to Gymboree when he could just sit up, crawl and walk and he enjoyed it each time.

Call for times when your child's age group meets.

5001 NE 50th Street, Laurelhurst	(206)522–2045
9250 14th Avenue NW, Crown Hill	(206)523–8011
2331 NE 140th Avenue, Bellevue	(425)392–8438
3302 E Lake Sammamish Parkway, Issaquah	(425)392–8438
33633 S 9th Avenue, Federal Way	(253) 661–7205

★★★
KINDERMUSIK BEGINNINGS
1–800–628–5687 for a location near you

Kindermusik International has developed a curriculum to introduce youngsters to the world of music. Kindermusik Beginnings is designed specifically for toddlers eighteen months to three and a half years old. For thirty minutes, once a week, both parent and child participate in singing, musical instrument exploration and movement.

These structured classes, developed by early childhood education and music specialists, are designed to be fun as well as educational. Freelance instructors are trained by Kindermusik International and hold classes in their homes. Kindermusik Beginnings classes are also offered at various community centers. Kindermusik International recommends an $85 fee per semester, although Kindermusik classes taught at community centers may be less expensive.

★★★★
PUBLIC LIBRARIES

Some libraries offer Toddler Storytime, Rock and Read, or Mother Goose Storytime—different names for storytime geared toward children under two. For half an hour a children's librarian or local volunteer reads stories aloud, and arts and crafts activities are sometimes offered. These storytimes are best for toddlers who can sit still. At fourteen months, my boy could not sit still during Toddler Storytime at the Green Lake Branch; however, others his age were quiet on their mother's laps.

Libraries on the Eastside also offer Toddler Time for children two to three years old. In Seattle, the public libraries offer storytimes during all months except May, September, and December. Always phone first for times and availability. Many of the public libraries have a children's books section that not only has books available for you to read to your child, but also has toys and puzzles set out to occupy youngsters.

Montlake Branch–Toddler Storytime (206)684–4720
2300 E 24th Avenue

Queen Anne Branch–Toddler Storytime (206)386–4227
400 W Garfield Street

Green Lake Branch–Toddler Storytime (206)684–7547
7364 E Green Lake Drive North

Northeast Branch–Toddler Storytime (206)684–7539
6801 NE 35th Avenue

Lake City Branch–Rock and Read (206)684–7518
12501 NE 28th Avenue

Multiple Locations

**Newport Way Library–Mother Goose Storytime
and Toddler Time** (425)747–2390
14250 SE Newport Way, Bellevue

Ballard–Toddler Storytime (206)684–4089
5711 NW 24th Avenue

Southwest Branch–Toddler Storytime (206)684–7455
9010 SW 35th Avenue

Holly Park Branch–Toddler Storytime (206)386–1905
6748 S 35th Avenue

West Seattle Branch–Toddler Storytime (206)684–7444
2306 SW 42nd Avenue

**Lake Hills Library–Mother Goose Storytime and
Toddler Time** (425)747–3350
15228 Lake Hills Boulevard

**Issaquah Library–Mother Goose Storytime and
Toddler Time** (425)392–5430
120 E Sunset Way

Bellevue Regional Library–Toddler Time (425)450–1775
1111 N 110th Avenue

Kirkland Public Library–Toddler Time (425)822–245
308 Kirkland Avenue

★★★★
BOOKSTORES

Many of the chain and independent bookstores have excellent children's departments filled with a wide variety of books for youngsters. They also have storytime available to children of all ages. There usually is not an age requirement for storytime; however, you need to be the judge of your own baby's ability to sit and listen. Fortunately, if your child gets restless you can get up and walk around and look at all the books available for purchase.

The following bookstores have storytimes for young children. Those that have a preferred age for their attendees are not listed here.

Barnes and Noble/Bellevue (425)451-8463
626 NE 106th Avenue, Bellevue

Barnes and Noble/Issaquah (425)557-8808
1530 NW 11th Avenue, Issaquah

Barnes and Noble/Southcenter (206)575-3965
300 W Andover Park, Tukwila 2

Barnes and Noble/University Village (206)517-4107
2700 NE University Village, Seattle

Borders Books/Redmond (425)869-1907
16549 NE 74th Street, Redmond

Borders Books/Seattle (206)622-4599
1501 Fourth Avenue, Seattle

Borders Books/Tukwila (206)575-4506
17501 Southcenter Parkway, Tukwila

Stars (425)392-2900
55 NE Gilman Boulevard, Issaquah

All for Kids Books and Music (206)526-2768
2900 NE Blakely Street, Seattle

University Bookstore (206)634-3400
4326 NE University Way, Seattle

Third Place Books (206)366–3333
17171 NE Bothell Way, Lake Forest Park

The Secret Garden (206)789–5006
6115 NW 15th Avenue, Ballard

★★★
PUBLIC SWIMMING POOLS

Swim lessons for babies and toddlers begin at four to six months old, and run up to three or four years old. This is a fine way to get your child accustomed to the water in a warm pool with other young children and parents. I found that the morning classes are filled with women and babies and the evening classes have mostly men with their children. The locker room floors can be cold, so be prepared. Most pools offer pay lockers and changing tables. Babies need swim diapers or cloth diapers with rubber diaper pants to prevent unwanted spills. Bring a polyester top to help keep your baby warm. When my child could not walk I brought my stroller, where he waited while we changed our clothes. Classes last half an hour and usually cost about $3-4 per class, with six to eight classes per session. Many of the pools have a family swim open to children of all ages, with no registration necessary.

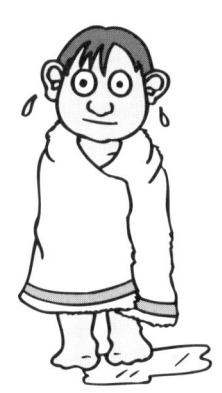

Ballard Pool (206)684–4094
1471 NW 67th Street, Ballard
  Evening classes available

Bellevue Aquatics Center (425)452–4444
601 NE 143rd Avenue, Bellevue
  Evening and weekend classes available

Coleman Pool (outdoors) (206)684–7494
8603 SW Fauntleroy Way, West Seattle

Evans Pool (206)684–4961
7201 E Green Lake Drive, Green Lake
    Evening and weekend classes available

Helene Madison Pool (206)684–4979
13401 N Meridian Avenue, Lake City
    Evening classes available

Issaquah's Julius Boehm Pool (425)837–3350
50 SE Clark Street, Issaquah

Meadowbrook Pool 206) 684–4989
10515 NE 35th Avenue, Lake City

Medgar Evers Pool (206)684–4766
500 E 23rd Avenue, Central
    Evening and weekend classes available

Mounger Pool (outdoors) (206)684–4708
2535 W 32nd Avenue, Magnolia
    Evening classes available

Peter Kirk Pool (outdoors) (425)828–1235
380 NE Kirkland Avenue, Kirkland

Queen Anne Aquatic Center (206)386–4282
1920 W 1st Avenue, Queen Anne
    Evening and weekend classes available

Rainier Beach Pool (206)386–1944
8825 S Rainier Avenue, South Seattle
    Evening and weekend classes available

Multiple Locations

Redmond City Pool (206)296-2961
17535 NE 104th Avenue NE, Redmond
   Evening classes available

Southwest Pool (206)684-7440
2801 SW Thistle, South Seattle
   Evening classes available

★★★
PRIVATE SWIMMING POOLS

As with public pools, private swimming pools or private lessons offer an excellent way for babies to get used to the water. The pools are kept warm and the class sizes are kept to a minimum. Prices vary and sometimes there is an additional registration or annual membership fee. Call for times and fees.

Ballard Olympic Athletic Club (206)706-4882
2208 NW Market, Ballard
   Offers tot swim for non-members.

Bellevue Family YMCA (425)746-9900
14230 Bel-Red Road, Bellevue

Kid Swim (206)364-7946
14540 NE Bothell Way, Lake City

Safe 'N Sound Swimming (206)285-9279
2040 N Westlake Avenue, Queen Anne

Waterbabies Aquatic Program (425)643-4334
1213 NE 162nd Lane, Bellevue
   Classes offered in Bellevue and Redmond.

Central Seattle

Central Seattle, the heart of the city, includes the neighborhoods of Capitol Hill, Madison Park, Queen Anne, Magnolia and Downtown Seattle. Parents will find an exciting range of things to do with their child, both indoors and out, in this busy section of the city. Here you will find three of the city's best known parks: Discovery Park, Volunteer Park and Washington Park Arboretum. For indoor recreation, the Children's Museum and Seattle Aquarium are easily accessible in the downtown area.

Indoor Activities

★★

BAY PAVILION CAROUSEL (206)623-8600

Pier 57, Alaskan Way, Downtown

Hours: Daily 11 a.m.–8 p.m.
Fees: $1 per child
Access: Lot or metered street parking (25¢ per 15 minutes, 2 hours maximum); stroller access
Weekend/evening hours: Yes
Features: Restrooms, food and drink

No changing table, no nursing privacy, no play equipment for tots

A carousel's colorful lights and sounds may stimulate a younger infant, but an actual ride is best for babies who can sit

Indoor Activities

up. My one-year-old enjoyed the merry-go-round ride and was not frightened by the music or movement. Summertime brings hordes of tourists to this area, so if you want a hassle-free visit, go during the winter on a weekday. I found the place empty on winter weekdays and we were allowed to ride as long as we wanted. Activity picks up in the evenings, and increases even more on weekends. On your way back to your car you will find the Seattle Sourdough Bakery, where you can pick up an excellent roll for the ride home, if your little one has started eating solids.

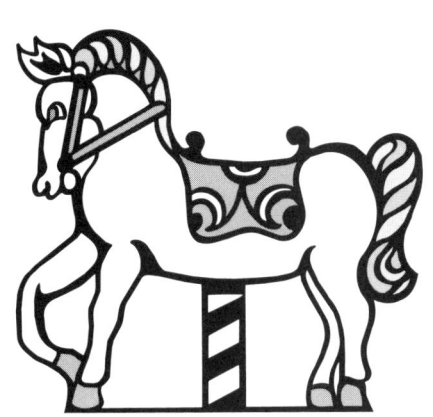

★★★½

CHILDREN'S MUSEUM (206)441–1768
Seattle Center House, Lower Level, Seattle

Hours: Monday–Friday 10 a.m.–5 p.m., Saturday and Sunday 10 a.m–6 p.m.; June 15 to Labor Day, Monday–Friday 10 a.m.–6 p.m, Saturday and Sunday 10 a.m.–7 p.m.
Fees: Children 2–12 $5.50, adults $4.00, annual pass $48
Access: Lot and street parking; stroller access
Classes: Offered mostly to children over three
Weekend/evening hours: Yes
Features: Play equipment for tots (see below), restrooms, changing table, food and drink (Food Pavilion upstairs)

No nursing privacy

The Children's Museum is designed for older infants, toddlers and older children. Two sections of the museum are re-creations of villages from different cultures throughout the world. Carpeted rooms to the left of the entry, which are relatively quiet and have playthings close to the ground, are good for crawlers. A special area with a slide and toys is reserved for children under two and a half. Craft time, available for older children, probably is not appropriate for your baby. Do not go during spring break as the museum fills up with older children who could intimidate a small toddler. The best value is buying a year's membership if you think you will go often.

COOPERATIVE PRESCHOOLS

See Multiple Locations, pages 23–24.

★★½

GARFIELD FAMILY CENTER   (206)461-4486

Garfield Community Center
2323 E Cherry Street, Central

Hours: Open Monday–Friday 9 a.m.–5 p.m.; call for class times
Access: Parking; stroller access
Classes: PEPS–Parent/Child Activity Time (0–3 years)
Weekend/evening hours: Yes
Features: Play equipment for tots, restrooms, changing table, nursing privacy, food and drink in vending machines, playground outside the center (see page 39)

This small room, furnished with toys and games for young children, is found as you enter the Garfield Community Center. A variety of classes for adults, families and teen parents are offered, and parent/tot drop-in is planned for the future. Call to get on their mailing list.
PEPS Parent/Child Activity Time. This activity group is open to parents with children under three

years old, although exceptions are made for siblings. Everyone is welcome at this special time which provides socialization for youngsters as well as support for parents. The meeting, which usually is offered on Wednesday afternoons, includes playtime and an informal, facilitator-led discussion with the parents. Children make crafts with their parents' help, and the youngsters' snack time is followed by singing and games.

★★★
MAGNOLIA COMMUNITY CENTER   (206)386–4235
2550 W 34th Avenue, Magnolia

Hours: Monday–Friday 10 a.m.–10 p.m. and Saturday 9 a.m.–5 p.m.; call for class times
Access: Parking; stroller access
Classes: Tot Gym (under 5 years), Tot Bop (1½–3½ years), Baby Bop (under 18 months)
Weekend/evening hours: Yes
Features: Restrooms (small), food and drink in vending machines, playground outside the center (see page 46)

No play equipment for tots, no changing table, no nursing privacy

The Magnolia Community Center is located next to a grade school. Since the center also has a preschool inside, the restroom must shared with a lot of three-year-olds

The center offers several options for those under three:

Baby Bop. For babies who are sitting and crawling but not walking. Forty-five minutes is devoted to music, songs and movements that you practice with your baby.

Tot Bop. Songs, music and props are used to get parents and toddlers moving about. It meets once a week for forty-five minutes.

Tot Gym. During this class the

gym is closed to everyone except parents and children. Unfortunately, no equipment or toys are provided by the center, so parents must bring their own. This program is ongoing.

★★★★
PACIFIC SCIENCE CENTER (206)443-2880
200 N Second Avenue, Seattle Center, Downtown

Hours: Summer 10 a.m.–6 p.m. daily; winter Monday–Friday 10 a.m.–5 p.m. and Saturday–Sunday 10 a.m.–6 p.m.
Fees: Adults 14–64 $7:50, children 6–13 and seniors 65+ $5:50, preschool 2–3 $3.50, under 2 free, annual pass $52
Access: Parking lots (fee) and street (metered); stroller access
Weekend/evening hours: Yes
Features: Play equipment for tots (see below), restrooms, changing table, nursing privacy, food and drink in Food Pavilion

The Pacific Science Center museum is primarily for older children, however it has a great play area available for toddlers and babies. In Building Two adequate space has been reserved for a popular play area. A large trough of water is filled with toys used for water play, a low maze is fun to explore, and plastic slides and climbers are on hand. Adjoining this space are two smaller rooms with more toys and a private nursing area.

The rest of the Pacific Science Center is filled with learning exhibits for adults and older children. The Food Pavilion, located on the Seattle Center grounds, offers a variety of foods.

Indoor Activities

★★★
REI DOWNTOWN STORE   (206)223-1944

222 N Yale Avenue, Downtown

Hours: Monday–Friday 10 a.m.–9 p.m., Saturday 9 a.m.–9 p.m., Sunday 11 a.m.–6 p.m.
Access: Garage parking (no charge) and street; stroller access
Weekend/evening hours: Yes
Features: Play equipment for tots (see below), restrooms, changing table, nursing privacy in women's restroom, food and drink at TODO Wraps concession

What a fun place to visit with your toddler! This huge store can be very exciting. Before entering the store your little ones can gaze at the waterfall outside. Then once inside they can see the giant fiberglass climbing rock, bronze animal tracks and an oversized glass compass embedded in the floor. Upstairs in the clothing section is a toddler play area. It is worth a visit just to browse, but if you need any type of sporting, camping or biking gear, REI is a great place to shop. Some clothes and shoes are available for older and larger infants. We bought our backpack child carrier and our bike trailer here. Ramps and elevators make stroller use easy, so you can bring your own stroller or use ones that REI provides for older babies. There is even a quiet nursing room in the women's restroom.

★★½
SEATTLE AQUARIUM   (206)386-4320

1483 Alaskan Way, (Pier 59 Waterfront Park), Downtown

Hours: Summer–daily 10 a.m.–7 p.m.; winter–daily 10 a.m.–5 p.m.
Fees: Adults $8.00, children 6–18 $5.25, children 3–5 $3.25, under 2 years free, seniors 65+ $7.00, annual pass $50; King County resident discounts
Access: Lot or metered street parking (25¢ per 15 minutes, 2 hours maximum); stroller access

Weekend/evening hours: Yes
Features: Restrooms, changing table, nursing privacy, food and drink nearby

No play equipment for tots

The Seattle Aquarium is a good place to take a baby old enough to sit in a stroller. The entire museum is ramped, making stroller use a breeze, and most of the fish tanks begin at floor level, so you can push the baby right up to the tank for close viewing. My infant enjoyed looking at all the different sizes and colors of fish. Sea mammals are housed in glass tanks that open up to the fresh air. Winter seems to hold the crowds down. Groups of children occasionally come for field trips during the school year; however, the aquarium is big enough for you to avoid these groups if you wish. I moved through the entire museum in an hour and a half with baby riding happily along in the stroller. The restroom farther into the aquarium has a handicap stall that will fit a stroller.

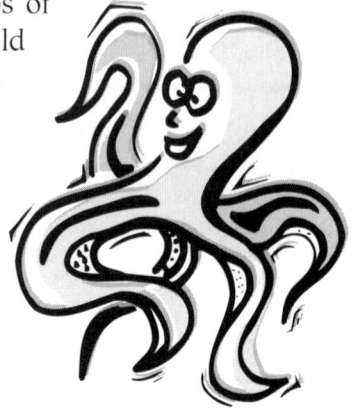

SEATTLE PUBLIC LIBRARIES: TODDLER STORYTIME

Queen Anne Branch, Montlake Branch; see Multiple Locations, pages 26–27.

SWIMMING POOLS: TOT SWIM

Medgar Evers Pool, Mounger Pool, Queen Anne Aquatic Center, Safe 'N Sound Swimming; see Multiple Locations, pages 29–31.

Outdoor Activities

Montlake, Madison Park, Capitol Hill & The Central Area

★½
GARFIELD COMMUNITY CENTER PARK   (206)461-4486
2323 Cherry Street E, Central

Access: Parking; stroller access
Features: Play equipment for tots (slides, swings, climbers, spinner), woodchip play area surface, restrooms, changing table, nursing privacy, food and drink in vending machines, some shade

This small playground is part of the Garfield Community Center. The play equipment may be a little sophisticated for toddlers, but the park can be used if you have been visiting the Garfield Family Center and want to take your child outside. Restrooms, changing table and vending machines are in the center.

★★★★
MADISON PARK
Madison Street and 42nd Avenue E, Madison Park

Access: Parking
Features: Play equipment for tots (slides, swings, climbers, bouncers, spinner), sand play area surface, restrooms by the beach, some nursing privacy, some shade

No stroller access, no changing table

This is an exciting park to visit with children of all ages. Toddlers can be kept busy with the play equipment, while infants will enjoy picking dandelions off the grassy field. Stop first for a bagel and coffee or other beverage from a neighborhood shop. A cool breeze often blows off Lake Washington on hot summer days, so you might want sweaters for you and your child. Just east of the playground is a beach with restrooms.

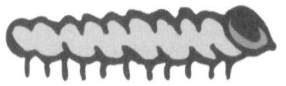

★★
ROANOKE PARK

Roanoke Street and Broadway E, Montlake

Access: Parking; stroller access
Features: Play equipment for tots (slides, swings, climbers), sand play area surface, some nursing privacy, some shade

No restrooms, no changing table, no food or drink

This pleasant neighborhood park lies nestled between the Highway 520 freeway and Interstate 5, making the noise factor high during rush hours. It is also right across the street from a fire station. If the noise potential does not deter you, this neighborhood is an attractive place in which to walk, and the park makes a nice resting spot.

★★★★
VOLUNTEER PARK   Wading pool hotline (206)684–7796

Prospect Street and 14th Avenue E, Capitol Hill

Access: Parking; stroller access
Features: Play equipment for tots (slides, swings, climbers, bouncers) sand play area surface, wading pool, restrooms, nursing privacy, shade

No changing table, no food or drink available

As you drive into Volunteer Park you will see a large brick

water tower. Continue on, passing the Asian Art Museum and reaching the top of the park. Stop here, get out the stroller, and walk to the greenhouse conservatory. Most of the beautiful plants and flowers on display here are low enough to permit good stroller viewing.

A short walk from the Conservatory is a large playground that offers a variety of equipment. The play area and round wading pool are partially shaded. Across from the playground is a large grassy field where you and your baby can stretch out and relax.

★★

WASHINGTON PARK ARBORETUM

*Lake Washington Boulevard and Madison Street E,
    Madison Park*

Access: Parking; jog stroller access
Features: Restrooms, nursing privacy, shade

No play equipment for tots, no changing table, no food or drink available

The Washington Park Arboretum is a large botanical preserve in the middle of Seattle's Montlake District. Winding trails take you through beds of a variety of beautiful flowers, and the gift shop is a pleasant stop. Bring a pack and a lunch and take the time to enjoy this bit of nature within the big city. There is a small play area in the lower area of the park and the walk over the bridge that spans Lake Washington Boulevard is very nice.

Queen Anne

★ ½

EAST QUEEN ANNE PARK

Wading pool hotline
(206)684-7796

Howe Street and 2nd Avenue W

Access: Parking; stroller access
Features: Play equipment for tots (swings), sand play area surface, wading pool, restrooms, some shade

No changing table, no nursing privacy, no food or drink available

This quaint neighborhood park holds a nice, slightly shaded wading pool. The playground is small, but is adequate for toddlers. This is a fine park to walk to for a short visit.

★★

MAYFAIR PARK

Raye Street and 2nd Avenue W

Access: Parking; stroller access
Features: Play equipment for tots (slide, climbers), sand play area surface, restrooms, nursing privacy, shade

No changing table, no food or drink available

This delightful park sits atop the eastern slope of Queen Anne Hill. Although play equipment is sparse, the peaceful setting makes up for what may be missing. This hidden park makes a fine retreat.

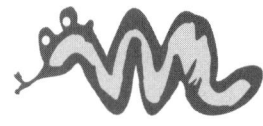

★★½
ROGERS PARK

Raye Street and 1st Avenue W

Access: Parking scarce—try 3rd Avenue; stroller access
Features: Play equipment for tots (slides, swings, climbers, spinner), woodchip play area surface, restrooms, nursing privacy, shade

No changing table, no food or drink available

The city of Seattle has recently built a new playground at Rogers Park, a large wooded area on the northern slope of Queen Anne hill. Parking is tight, so the park is best for those visitors who live within walking distance. Trees provide the shade and privacy needed for mothers of very young infants.

★★★
WEST QUEEN ANNE PARK

Howe Street and 3rd Avenue W

Access: Parking; stroller access
Features: Play equipment for tots (slides, swings, climbers, spinner), sand play area surfaces, restrooms in community center, little shade

No changing table, no food or drink available, no nursing privacy

This playground in the center of Queen Anne Hill offers play equipment appropriate for toddlers and older children. Since it is near a middle school, you might want to avoid the park during lunchtime and after school. I went when classes were in session and the playground was empty. The community center about fifty yards to the east doesn't have activities for babies, but there is a restroom in the building. Restaurants can be found on Queen Anne Boulevard, a few blocks away.

Magnolia

★★½

BAYVIEW PARK

Armour Street and 24th Avenue W

Access: Parking; stroller access
Features: Play equipment for tots (slide, swings, climbers), sand play area surface, restrooms, moderate shade

No changing table, no food or drink available, no nursing privacy

This small park is found in a quiet Magnolia neighborhood. The playground is above the playfield and is well shaded. Parking is on the streets surrounding the park.

★★½

DISCOVERY PARK

Commodore Way and 40th Avenue W

Access: parking; stroller access
Features: Restrooms, nursing privacy, shade

No stroller access, no play equipment for tots, no changing table, no food or drink available

If you like to hike, but do not want to drive out of the city, this park is for you. Trails ramble throughout the wooded preserve. One of the best trails runs through a wooded incline and along a ridge overlooking Puget Sound. Lush meadows invite resting and picnicking. Bring your back carrier because strollers will not work well on the dirt trails. Be careful if you let your toddler walk along the trail as there are some drop-off points along the bluff. Check out the visitor's center and ask about the toddler nature walks.

★★½
LAWTON PARK

Thurman Street and 26th Avenue W

Access: Parking on 26th Avenue; stroller access
Features: Play equipment for tots (slides, swings, climbers, spinner), sand play area surface, some nursing privacy, some shade

No restrooms, no changing table, no food or drink available

Terraced Lawton Park is built into the northern slope of Magnolia Bluff, overlooking Ballard. A small playground is located above Lawton School in the middle of a hilly, forested park. A paved pathway leads up to the playground, and wooded trails go deeper into the park. When parking on 26th Avenue, park by the pathway, not by the school's private playground. You may also park on Williams Avenue and take the path to the park.

★★½
MAGNOLIA PARK

Clise Place and Galer Avenue W

Access: Parking on street; stroller access
Features: Restrooms, nursing privacy, shade

No play equipment for tots, no changing table, no food or drink available

This beautiful piece of land is located on the western bluff of Magnolia. Although no play equipment is available, picnic benches are plentiful. To the west is a magnificent view of Puget Sound. Magnolia Park is easily accessed from the Magnolia Bridge.

★★
WEST MAGNOLIA PLAYGROUND

2550 W 34th Avenue

Access: Parking; stroller access

Features: Play equipment for tots (slide, swings, climbers, spinner), sand play area surface, restrooms, food and drink on McGraw Avenue, some shade

No changing table, no nursing privacy

This very popular park has enough equipment available to keep every youngster busy, although the slides may be a bit too difficult for some toddlers to negotiate. The playground rests below the community center, preventing children from running into the street. A grassy field adjacent to the playground is perfect for the non-walking child. Restrooms and vending machines are in the community center, but for coffee and food try McGraw Avenue.

See the Magnolia Community Center description, pages 35–36.

NORTH SEATTLE

Parks and playgrounds are plentiful in North Seattle; popular Green Lake Park and the Woodland Park Zoo are landmarks. This section of Seattle includes the northeast neighborhoods of Laurelhurst, Green Lake, Wallingford, Lake City and View Ridge, among others, and the northwest neighborhoods of Ballard, Fremont, Phinney Ridge, Loyal Heights and Crown Hill. Shoreline, a city north of Seattle, is also included in this chapter.

Indoor Activities

ALL FOR KIDS BOOKS AND MUSIC: STORYTIME

See Multiple Locations, pages 27–28.

★★★★
ALL THAT DANCE (206)524-8944

5507 NE 35th Avenue, Laurelhurst

Access: Parking; stroller access
Hours and fees: Call for times and fees
Classes: Toddler Creative Movement (2–4 years)
Weekend/evening hours: Nothing offered for tots
Features: Restrooms, food and drink nearby

No play equipment for tots, no changing table, no nursing privacy

In these classes, a small group of children two to four years old, with their parents, gathers together for movement, dancing and songs. This lightly-structured class offers an opportunity for youngsters to get accustomed to dancing and dance studios.

★★★★
BALLARD COMMUNITY CENTER (206)684-4093
6020 NW 28th Avenue, Ballard

Access: Parking; stroller access
Hours and fees: Monday–Friday 10 a.m.–10 p.m. and Saturday 9 a.m.–3 p.m.; call for class times and fees
Classes: Toddler Play Room (under 4 years); Gym Tot Time (under 5 years); Fun With Friends (2–3 years); Morning Step It Up Aerobics
Weekend/evening hours: Yes, playroom may open on Saturdays
Features: Play equipment for tots (playground page 83, restrooms, food and drink in vending machines

No changing table, no nursing privacy

Toddler Play Room. The center has turned its game room into a toddler room replete with riding toys, books, mats and a slide. Although it is a little small, it does not get too crowded, and provides an enjoyable place to play and meet others.

Tot Drop. The center opens its gym for children of all ages, with their parents, to run and play providing balls and mats. Parents are welcome to bring their own playthings. This arrangement is perfect for groups that don't want to offer their living rooms as meeting places, but still want to get together. When I visited the center there were about twenty two- to three-year-olds.

Fun with Friends. This class provides an opportunity for learning and socializing. You can drop off your two-year-old for singing, playing and making arts and crafts.

Morning Step It Up Aerobics. Childcare is available for mothers taking this one hour low-impact aerobics class.

See the Ballard Community Center playground description, page 830.

★★★½
BALLARD FAMILY CENTER (206)706–9645

5449 NW Ballard Avenue, Ballard

Access: Parking; stroller access
Hours and fees: Monday 1–5 p.m., Tuesday–Thursday 10 a.m.–5 p.m., Friday 10 a.m.–3 p.m.; call for class times and fees
Classes: Playroom (all ages); Kindermusik (0–18 months); Music and Storytime (all ages); Moms on the Move (infants); PEPS Parent/Child Activity Time (0–3 years)
Features: Play equipment for tots (see below), restrooms, changing table, food and drink nearby, nursing privacy

Located in the heart of the Ballard shopping district, this family center has plenty of activities for children under three.

Playroom. The small playroom is open at various times during the week for drop-in playtime. Toys and books are available for your child.

Kindermusik. These classes are a fine way to introduce your baby to music.

Music and Storytime. Singing, finger play and listening to music are the focus of this activity group.

Moms on the Move. This post-partum and pre-natal aerobics class for moms and their babies and is a great way to get back to exercising after having your baby.

Parent/Child Activity Time. This two-hour activity group is open to parents with children under three years old, although exceptions are made for siblings. The group begins with playtime while the facilitator leads an informal discussion with the parents. Snacks, crafts and singing are also part of the program.

★★★
BALLARD OLYMPIC ATHLETIC CLUB (206)789–5010
5301 Leary NW Avenue, Ballard

Access: Parking; stroller access
Hours and fees: Health club is open 24 hours a day except Saturday and Sunday; call for class times and fees
Classes: Moms and More Aerobics (babies in car seats, or additional fee for childcare). Tot Swim, see page 31.
Weekend/evening hours: Yes
Features: Play equipment for tots in daycare only, restrooms, changing table, food and drink, nursing privacy

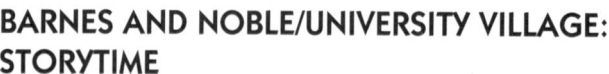

Mothers do not have to be members of the athletic club to enroll in their low-impact aerobics class, and they are encouraged to bring their babies if they are not crawling. When I visited, infants in car seats lined the mirrored walls as their mothers worked off unwanted pounds. Mothers with toddlers and crawling babies are encouraged to leave the children with competent caregivers in the nursery on the first floor.

This is a fully equipped health club with a great deal to offer in addition to aerobics. Stop by for a tour of the facilities if membership interests you.

BARNES AND NOBLE/UNIVERSITY VILLAGE: STORYTIME

See Multiple Locations, pages 27–28.

★★½
BITTER LAKE COMMUNITY CENTER (206)684–7524
13035 N Linden Avenue, Bitter Lake

Access: Parking; stroller access
Hours: Monday–Thursday 9 a.m.–9 p.m., Friday 9 a.m.–6 p.m.,

Saturday 9 a.m.–5 p.m.; call for class times and fees
Classes: Toddler Open Gym (under 5 years); Discovery Corner Juniors (2–3½ years)
Weekend/evening hours: Nothing offered for tots
Features: Play equipment for tots (see below), restrooms, changing table, food and drink in vending machines

No nursing privacy

This new community center opened in the spring of 1997.

Toddler Open Gym. The center provides balls, scarves, a tunnel, small hoops, and a mat for tumbling. The gym is open to toddlers for two hours, twice a week.

Discover Corner Juniors. For two hours your child is provided with crafts, stories and gym play. This is a scaled-down preschool for 2–3 year-olds. The emphasis is on social skills, cooking, science, art projects, singing and reading. A maximum of ten children participate with a teacher and a helper; parents are not required to stay.

See the Bitter Lake Park description, page 73.

★★★
BITTER LAKE FAMILY CENTER (206)368-0172
13035 N Linden Avenue, Bitter Lake

Access: Parking; stroller access
Hours: Monday, Tuesday, Thursday, Friday 12–5 p.m., Wednesday and Saturday 9 a.m.–5 p.m., Friday 10 a.m.–3 p.m. (some classes held in the evenings)
Classes: Drop-In PlayTime (all ages); PEPS Parent/child Activity Time (0–3 years)
Weekend/evening hours: Yes
Features: Play equipment for tots (see below), restrooms, changing table, nursing privacy, food and drink

This family center located in the Bitter Lake Community Center offers some activities for babies. The hours change quarterly, so call before you come.

Drop-In PlayTime. Caregivers are welcomed to bring their child to play in the playroom at different times during the week. There are scheduled times that the playroom is open but you can also use the playroom any time it is not being used for childcare.

Parent/Child Activity Time. This two-hour activity group is open to parents with children under three years old, although exceptions are made for siblings. The group begins with playtime for the children, while the facilitator leads an informal discussion with the parents. Snacks, crafts and singing are also a part of the program.

★★★★
CAMEO DANCE (206)528-8183

6560 NE Latona Avenue, Green Lake

Access: Parking; stroller access
Hours and fees: Call for times and fees
Classes: Parent/Toddler (2–3½ years)
Weekend/evening hours: Not for tots
Features: Restrooms, food and drink nearby, nursing privacy in a comfortable lobby

No play equipment for tots, no changing table

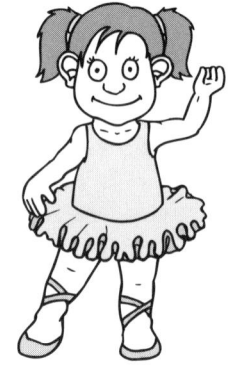

The Parent/Toddler class offered by this center is a fine introduction to dance. Youngsters are taught basic and creative dance movement. Ribbons and other props are used while children move to live music. The class meets once a week for forty-five minutes.

COOPERATIVE PRESCHOOLS

See Multiple Locations, pages 23–24.

★★★★
CREATIVE DANCE CENTER (206)363-7281

12577 N Densmore Avenue, Haller Lake

Access: Parking; stroller access
Hours and fees: Call for times and fees
Classes: Parent/Toddler (1½ –3 years); Parent/Infant (3 months– 14 months)
Weekend/evening hours: Yes
Features: Restrooms

No play equipment for tots, no changing table, no food or drink available, no nursing privacy

In classes at the Creative Dance Center parents and children use music, props and instruments to explore movement and dance. The hour-long class is designed to be fun as well as educational. The Haller Lake location is in the same building as the Haller Lake Community Club. The Phinney Ridge location is in the Phinney Neighborhood Center at 6532 North Phinney Avenue.

★★★★
DANCE FREMONT (206)633-0812

900 N 34th Street, Fremont

Access: Parking; stroller access
Hours and fees: Call for time and class fee
Classes: Parent/Toddler (2–3 years)
Features: Play equipment for tots (see below), restrooms

No changing table, no food or drink available, no nursing privacy

The instructor at Dance Fremont is a developmental specialist and involves parents and children in movement, dance, props and singing. The class is currently for two and three-year-olds but she may lower the age requirement to eighteen months. Located just east of the Aurora Bridge on North 34th Street, the studio is easy to miss if you don't watch carefully for it.

★★★½
FAMILY WORKS (206)694-6727
1501 N 45th Avenue, Wallingford

Access: Parking; stroller access
Hours: Monday–Friday 9 a.m.–5 p.m.; call for class times
Classes: Drop-In Playtime (0–5 years); Drop-In Storytime (2–5 years); Spanish for Toddlers; Parent/Child Activity Time (under 3 years)
Features: Play equipment for tots (see below), restrooms, changing table, food and drink nearby

No nursing privacy

Family Works moved into this new building in 1998. All the offerings are free.

Drop-In Playtime. Toys, Legos® and books are provided in a clean, carpeted room perfect for rainy days. Babies can intermingle with toddlers without the threat of being run over by a rolling toy. This room is usually open Fridays 9 a.m.–11 a.m.

Spanish for Toddlers. Introduce your toddler to Spanish. This popular class fills up quickly.

Drop-In Storytime. For an hour, the Wallingford children's librarian reads stories and entertains toddlers.

Parent/Child Activity Time. Program for Early Parent Support (PEPS) sponsors this loosely-structured play group for children under three, although older siblings are welcome. The meeting begins with open playtime in a large room with tables, chairs and toys. A smaller adjacent room also has toys and games. The facilitator leads an informal discussion with the parents as the children play, then crafts

are made with the parents' help. A snack for the youngsters is followed by singing.

This class is great for families with more than one child. It is also handy for mothers who are continuing their regular PEPS meetings with older babies and do not want to volunteer their house to a group of active toddlers, and for mothers who want to get out and meet other moms. It is usually offered Thursdays at 10 a.m. No registration is necessary.

★★★
GREEN LAKE COMMUNITY CENTER (206)684–4961
7201 E Green Lake Drive, Green Lake

Access: Parking (busy); stroller access
Hours and fees: Monday–Friday 10 a.m.–10 p.m. and Saturday 9 a.m.–5 p.m.; call for class times and fees
Classes: Toddler Play Center (under 5 years); Morning Joggers/ Aerobics Babysitting (under 5 years); Storytelling (under 5 years)
Weekend/evening hours: Yes
Features: Play equipment for tots (see playground, pages 70–71), restrooms, changing table, food and drink in vending machines
No nursing privacy

Toddler Play Center. This playroom is open during most of the center's hours of operation. It is an advantage to have a playroom available almost all the time, but this one can feel small if there are too many children present. Toys for climbing, riding, rolling and hugging fill up this second-floor room. Some of the toys are broken and dirty, but new ones are introduced often. I did not like taking a pre-walker here because of the numerous older children running around and grabbing toys. A small riding toy that rolls down a track into the play area can pose a danger to babies. On rainy winter days the room is filled with children under five. Despite its flaws, this play center is useful when you absolutely have to get out of the house.

Morning Joggers/Aerobics Babysitting. Leave your child

in the playroom with a childcare giver for an hour and jog around the lake or take aerobics. Call for availability. This service is subject to change.

Storytelling. Twice a month a local storyteller tells stories to children under five-years-old.

See the Green Lake Park description, pages 70–71.

★★½

GUILD 45th STREET THEATER/ CRYING ROOM (206)633-3353

2115 N 45th Avenue, Wallingford

Access: No parking; stroller access
Fees: Before 6 p.m. Adults–$7.50; seniors, children and matinee–$4.25
Weekend/evening hours: Yes
Features: No play equipment for tots, restrooms, food and drink, nursing privacy

No changing table

Guild 45th Street Theater has a small crying room in its second theater. This older theater venue usually shows art-house movies and foreign films. The theater is ideal for small, sleeping infants, as the films usually are not loud or violent. Unfortunately, parking is tight.

GYMBOREE

See Multiple Locations, pages 24-25.

★★★

LAURELHURST COMMUNITY CENTER (206)684-7529

4554 NE 41st Street, Laurelhurst

Access: Parking; stroller access
Hours: Monday–Friday 9 a.m.–8.pm.; call for class times

Classes: Toddler Playroom (under 5 years); Toddler Art Play Group (2–3 years)
Features: Play equipment for tots (see playground, page 79), restrooms, food and drink in vending machines

No changing table, no nursing privacy

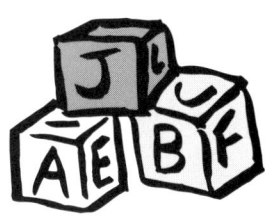

Toddler Playroom. The center's main room is filled with clean equipment for climbing and riding. There are mats in the center of the room but there is also uncovered wood flooring for rolling around in play cars. Toddler Playroom time is open for children under five; however, I did not see any children there over three. This is a good place for parents to come with a toddler and an infant. The playroom is usually open only on Friday mornings.

Toddler Art Play Group. For two hours in the morning, twice a week, you can leave your two year-old to have fun with paint, clay, drawing materials and more. This class is a good precursor to preschool. Along with focusing on art, the children are allowed to play with the center's toys. Music and reading are also offered. Two parents are required to assist each week, but most parents tend to stay anyway.

See the Laurelhurst Playground description, page 79.

★★★★
THE LITTLE GYM (206)524–2623

7777 15th Avenue NE, Lake City
Other locations: 1800 NE 130th Avenue, Bellevue,
  (425)885–3866; 4636 East Marginal Way, Georgetown,
  (206)524-2623

Access: Parking; stroller access
Hours and fees: Call for class times and fees
Classes: Bugs (4–10 months), Birds (10–19 months), Beasts (1½–2½ years)

Weekend/evening hours: Yes
Features: Play equipment for tots (see below), restrooms, changing table, food and drink at espresso cart

No nursing privacy

This gym's loosely structured classes offer toddlers and infants a chance to run, crawl, climb and bounce on various colorful pieces of equipment. At the beginning of the class the instructor sings a welcome song as parents and babies sing and dance in a circle. Free time comes next, giving children an opportunity to explore the equipment. The teacher guides the participants in the best ways to use the equipment to promote the baby's development. After free play, everyone gathers for more singing around the large multicolored parachute spread on the floor. Ball playing and then bubble blowing follow the parachute activity. The class ends with a goodbye song. I find these classes very stimulating for babies. There is not much interaction between the children, which is reassuring during cold season.

★★★★
LOYAL HEIGHTS COMMUNITY CENTER   (206)684–4052

2101 NW 77th Street, Loyal Heights

Access: Parking; no stroller access
Hours and fees: Monday–Friday 10 a.m.–10 p.m. and Saturday 9 a.m.–2:45 p.m.; call for class times and fees
Classes: Play Center–Co-op Young Preschooler (2½–3½ years); Play Center–Friday Night Co-op (1½–3½years); Play Center–Co-op Toddler (1–2½ years); Parent/Child Playgroup–Infant/Toddler (infants–24 months); Parent/Child Playgroup–Young Preschooler–(2–3½ years); Terrific Two's (2–3 years); Parent/Child Playgroup–Infants (infants–14 months); Parent/Child Playgroup–Mixed Ages (infants–3½ years); Parent/Child Playgroup–Evening (infants–3½ years); Drop-In Afternoons (infants–3½ years)
Weekend/evening hours: Yes

Features: Play equipment for tots (see playground, page 88), restrooms, changing table

No food or drink available, no nursing privacy

Play Center Co-op Classes. These classes include a structured time for playing, circle time and other activities. Parents are required to stay one day a week, but no other duties are required. Classes for older children have more structure than those for younger toddlers. The Friday Night Co-op enables parents to have one evening out every other Friday. Parents are required to stay a couple evenings in the semester.

Parent/Child Playgroup Classes. This is an excellent place for your child to explore different toys and equipment as well as to socialize in a safe environment. For ninety minutes parents and children gather for this informal class. During the first half of the class the children are free to wander about the room playing with toys designed for different ages. Then parents and children gather together for singing. The equipment and toys are clean and safe; everyone is friendly and relaxed.

Terrific Two's. This is a ninety-minute cooperative playtime for a maximum of five toddlers. The children are provided toys, activities, crafts and music. Parents are required to share duties and care.

Drop-In Afternoons. The playroom is open for unsupervised play. Parents are required to stay.

See the Loyal Heights Playground description, page 88.

★★½
MEADOWBROOK COMMUNITY CENTER (206)684–7522

10515 NE 35th Avenue, Lake City

Access: Parking; stroller access
Hours: Monday–Friday 9 a.m.–9:30 p.m. and Saturday 9 a.m.–5 p.m.; call for class times
Classes: Preschool Open Gym (under 5 years)
Weekend/evening hours: Nothing offered for tots

Features: Play equipment for tots (see below) restrooms, food and drink in vending machines

No changing table, no nursing privacy

The new community center at Meadowbrook is attached to the old swimming pool building. For two hours, twice a week, the center opens its large gym for children and parents to bring scooters, balls and other toys for play. Currently, the facility provides only mats, balls and a few other pieces of equipment. This arrangement is best for walkers and crawlers, and most of the children are under three. Expect to share your toys since toddlers don't know the meaning of "yours" and "mine." The availability of the open gym varies, so call for times.

★★½

MEADOWBROOK FAMILY CENTER   (206)366-9256

10517 NE 35th Avenue, Lake City
Access: Parking; stroller access
Hours: Monday–Friday 9 a.m.–5 p.m.; call for class times
Classes: Playroom (under 5 years); PEPS–Parent/Child Activity Time (under 3 years)
Features: Play equipment for tots (see below), restrooms, changing table, food and drink in vending machines, nursing privacy

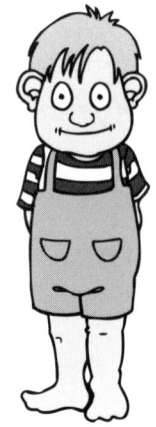

Located in the Meadowbrook Community Center on the second floor, this center has a small playroom with a variety of toys. It is usually open during the Family Center's hours of operation but times may vary in the summer. Offerings are free.

Parent/Child Activity Time. On Thursdays, for two hours, PEPS sponsors this special time in the playroom. It is open to parents with children under three years old, although exceptions are made for siblings. The meeting includes free playtime and an informal facilitator-led discussion for the parents. Children make crafts with their parents' help, are served a snack and then join together for singing. Everyone is welcome to this special time, which provides socialization for youngsters as well as support for parents.

★★

METRO CINEMAS/CRYING ROOM   (206)633-0055

4500 NE 9th Avenue, University District

Access: Parking lot with 1-hour validation; stroller access, elevator
Fees: Adults–$7.50, children and matinee–$4.25
Weekend/evening hours: Yes
Features: No play equipment for tots, restrooms, food and drink, nursing privacy

No changing table,

The exterior of this multiplex would lead you to believe it is one large theater. However, the building houses about ten small screens. The crying room, which is adequate, is in the rear of the theater. This movie theater screens many light comedies or family-oriented shows. Lack of parking and heavy traffic lessens the appeal of this movie theater.

★★

NORTHGATE THEATER/CRYING ROOM   (206)363–5800

10 Northgate Plaza (North end of Northgate Mall), Northgate

Access: Parking; stroller access
Fees: Before 6 p.m. Adults–$7; seniors, children and matinee–$4
Weekend/evening hours: Yes
Features: Restrooms, food and drink, nursing privacy

No play equipment for tots, no changing table

This is a one-screen movie theater that has an enclosed crying room far in the back . It is an older theater with cement floors and carpet only on the aisles. Crying rooms are great for younger infants who do not watch the screen. The theater often shows noisy, action-packed movies.

★★
NORTH SEATTLE FAMILY SUPPORT CENTER (206)364-7930

13540 NE Lake City Way, Suite 5, Lake City

Access: Parking limited; no stroller access
Fees: Monday–Friday 9 a.m.–5 p.m.; call for class times
Classes: PEPS–Parent/Child Activity Time (under 3 years)
Features: Play equipment for tots (see below), restrooms, changing table, snacks provided, nursing privacy

Parent/Child Activity Time. This two-hour activity group is open to parents with children under three, although exceptions are made for siblings. The group starts with open playtime in a large, carpeted room with toys, games and books available for younger children. A facilitator leads an informal discussion with parents, after which crafts are made with the parents' help. A snack served to the youngsters is followed by singing. The class is informal, so don't worry if you are late.

Parent/Child Activity Time is excellent for families with more than one child. It is also good for those moms who are continuing their regular PEPS meetings with their older babies, but do not want to volunteer their house to a group of active toddlers.

★★★★
RAVENNA-ECKSTEIN COMMUNITY CENTER (206)684-7534

6535 NE Ravenna Avenue, Ravenna

Access: Parking; stroller access
Hours and fees: Monday–Friday 9 a.m.–10 p.m., Saturday 9

Indoor Activities

a.m.–5 p.m.; call for class times and fees

Classes: Indoor Playspace Drop-In Center (under 5 years); Music Exploration (2–3 years); Ooey Gooey Play (2–3 years); Storytime (2 yr.); Toddler Open Gym (under 5 years) Tiny Tots (2–3 years and 2½–3½ years)

Weekend/evening hours: Yes

Features: Play equipment for tots (see below), restrooms, changing table, food and drink in vending machines

No nursing privacy

Indoor Playspace. A good-sized room contains pieces of large equipment and many toys. I went at 3 p.m. and found about five toddlers; by 4:30 there must have been over twenty. The toys and equipment were in good condition and clean, the room is carpeted and there are mats, especially around the plastic slide. The hours that this room is open varies; call for times.

Music Exploration. A maximum of ten toddlers with their parents join together for forty-five minutes, experimenting with musical instruments, singing, listening and moving their bodies. This class is not always offered.

Ooey Gooey Play. Toddlers spend forty-five minutes playing with different types of squishy materials such as Silly Putty and homemade playdough. This class is not always offered.

Storytime. The Seattle Public Library sponsors this storybook reading by a children's librarian.

Tiny Tots. For two hours, twice a week, you can leave your two-to-three-year old with an instructor and other children of a similar age. The maximum group size is twelve. Games, storytelling, arts and crafts are provided for entertainment. Parents are expected to assist with class duties several times during the session.

★★★★
SEATTLE GYMNASTICS ACADEMY   (206)362-7447
12535 NE 26th Avenue, Lake City

Access: Parking; stroller access
Hours and fees: Call for times and fees
Classes: Parent/Tot Class (18 months–3 years), Mommy and Me Fitness (infants in car seats)
Weekend/evening hours: Yes
Features: Play equipment for tots (see below), restrooms, food and drink in vending machines

No changing table, no nursing privacy

The Seattle Gymnastics Academy is designed for all levels of gymnastics, and for participants of all ages. The main room is filled with uneven bars, balance beams, trampolines and apparatuses used to train competitive gymnasts. In the rear, a smaller room used for the Parent/Tot class has soft tumbling objects perfect for toddlers. Also, there is a small nook near the bleachers you can use for babies who have siblings in other classes.

Parent/Tot Class. Although this class is open to children eighteen to thirty-six months, Most toddlers I saw were twenty-four months and up. These youngsters had no problem with sitting in a circle and following simple movements. I found that my twenty-one month old boy was not mature enough for this class, as he just wanted to run around and explore the equipment. The class begins with singing and bubble blowing. The children then sit in a circle for a short movement game. Then the toddlers are given time to explore the equipment. They are also brought into the large gym where they can play on the trampoline and other apparatuses. Toward the end of the class they jump into a pit filled with foam rubber blocks—it's hard to describe the activity, but the children enjoyed it.

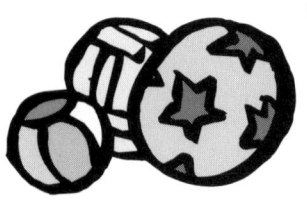

The academy is ideal for parents

with slightly older children as well as toddlers, as a class for four and five year olds is offered concurrently. If you wish to encourage your child to be involved in gymnastics, this is an ideal place to start.

Mommy and Me Fitness. Aerobics for pregnant and postpartum women.

SEATTLE PUBLIC LIBRARIES: TODDLER STORYTIME

Green Lake Branch, Northeast Branch, Lake City Branch, Ballard Branch, see Multiple Locations, pages 26–27.

★★★

THE SECRET GARDEN (206)789-5060

6115 NW 15th Avenue, Ballard

Access: Parking; stroller access
Hours and fees: Monday–Saturday 10 a.m.–6 p.m., Thursday 10 a.m.–8 p.m., Sunday 1–5 p.m.
Classes: Storytime (any age)
Weekend/evening hours: Yes
Features: Play equipment for tots (see below), restrooms

No changing table, no food or drink, no privacy for nursing

This bookstore provides a delightful alternative to large chain bookstores or public libraries. Convenient angled parking in front of the store allows you to whisk your baby from the car to the store in no time at all. Once inside you can seat your toddler at the low puzzle table to read books or play with puzzles and games while you rock your infant in a nearby comfortable rocker. There are enough nooks to provide for private nursing, and the bathroom is large enough to lay your changing pad on the floor to change a diaper. The store's knowledgeable staff can help find books suitable for your baby.

★★½
SHORELINE CENTER GYM   (206)546-5041

185th Street and 1st Avenue, Shoreline

Access: Parking; stroller access
Hours and fees: Call for times and fees
Classes: Indoor Playground (under 5 years), not offered in the summer
Features: Play equipment for tots (see below), restrooms

No changing table, no food or drink available, no nursing privacy

    This large gym contains toys and equipment for youngsters of varying ages. Unfortunately, the center does not open its gym for Indoor Playground during the summer months, so call ahead for times and dates. The Shoreline Center is a large complex of buildings just off 1st Avenue NE. The gym is behind the Center's auditorium on the eastern side of the complex.

★★½
SHORELINE FAMILY SUPPORT CENTER   (206)362-7282

17018 NE 15th Avenue, Shoreline

Access: Parking; no stroller access
Hours and fees: Monday–Friday 9 a.m.–5 p.m.; call for class times and fees
Classes: Indoor Playground (under 5 years)
Features: Play equipment for tots (see below), restrooms, changing table

No nursing privacy, no food or drink available

    The support center opens its preschool room to children under five years old for two hours on Friday. The room is small but it has numerous small toys and games. A low table with chairs is available for reading or crafts.

Indoor Activities

SWIMMING POOLS: TOT SWIM

Ballard Pool, Evans Pool, Helene Madison Pool, Meadowbrook Pool, Kid's Swim, Ballard Olympic Athletic Club; see Multiple Locations, pages 29–31.

★★★
TOP TEN TOYS (206)782-0098

104 N 85th Street, Crown Hill

Access: Parking; stroller access
Hours: Open Wednesday–Friday 9 a.m.–9 p.m. and Saturday–Tuesday 9 a.m.–6 p.m. (hours vary by the season)
Weekend/evening hours: Yes
Features: Play equipment for tots (toys for play and sale), restrooms, food and drink at nearby McDonalds, changing table, nursing privacy

This is not just an ordinary toy store. In addition to having every toy imaginable for all ages of children, there is also an area near the toddler section that has toys for your child to try out. You can see if your baby responds to the toy before purchasing it. The family restroom has a comfortable changing table and child-size toilet for potty-trained children.

★★★★
TUNE TALES (425)775-0608

John's Music, 4501 N Interlake, Wallingford. Other locations at Terrace Village, 2202 W 64th Avenue, Suite #2C, Mountlake Terrace; Home of Tune Tales, 7800 SW 185th Place, Edmonds

Access: Parking on street; stroller access
Hours and fees: Call for times and fees
Classes: Allegros (18 months–_3 years)
Features: Play equipment for tots (see below), restrooms, food and drink at Bagels on 45th Street
No changing table, no nursing privacy

Sign your toddler up for an enjoyable half hour of musical

fun. Two animated leaders engage the children by combining old favorite songs and new ones with musical instruments, teddy bears, scarves and more. The children are encouraged to participate with the props and are not pressured stay on their parent's lap. This is a great way to introduce your toddler to music.

UNIVERSITY BOOKSTORE: STORYTIME

See Multiple Locations, pages 27–28.

★★★★
UNIVERSITY FAMILY YMCA   (206)524–1400

5003 NE 12th Avenue, University District

Access: Parking; stroller access
Hours and fees: Monday–Friday 6 a.m.–10 p.m., Saturday 8 a.m.–5 p.m., Sunday 12–5 p.m.; call for class times and fees
Classes: Baby Fit (6–18 months); Parent/Tot (18–36 months); Aerobics for Moms (bring your baby to watch while you workout)
Weekend/evening hours: Yes
Features: Play equipment for tots (see below), restrooms, changing table

No nursing privacy, no food or drink available

Baby Fit. During Baby-Fit classes the gym is filled with large, colorful tumbling equipment. The forty-five-minute class is unstructured for about twenty minutes, then the instructor gathers everyone together for singing. The equipment is similar to Gymboree and Little Gym but there is no parachute or "Gymbo doll." Also, the cost is much less.

There is a registration fee in addition to the class fee.

Aerobics for Moms. For forty-five minutes you can take your under-three-year old with you to this aerobics class. The YMCA provides toys and mats in one corner of the gym for the little ones while mom works out.

Outdoor Activities & Beaches

Green Lake, Wallingford & Ravenna

★★
COWEN PARK

Ravenna Boulevard and 15th Avenue NE, Ravenna

Access: Parking; stroller access
Features: Play equipment for tots (slides, swings) woodchip play area surface, restrooms, nursing privacy, shade

No changing table, no food or drink available

A newly-built playground graces the southeast corner of this park. Cowen Park is actually an extension of Ravenna Park; both are situated along a wooded ravine. A smattering of picnic tables dapple the inner regions of the park where it intertwines with its sister and becomes one large play area. There is enough shade for comfort and plenty of places to bask in the warmth of an April sun. The woods between Cowen Park and Ravenna Park is a hangout for homeless teenagers.

★★½
GAS WORKS PARK

Northlake Way and Burke Avenue NE, Wallingford

Access: Parking; stroller access
Features: Play equipment for tots (slides, climbers, spinner), sand play area surface, restrooms, food and drink at concession stand, nursing privacy, some shade

No changing table

Gas Works Park has a gorgeous view of Lake Union and downtown Seattle. This old plant turned coal and oil into gas up until 1956. The rusted old gas pipes and pumps rising out of the ground now serve as a memorial to days gone by. A covered section contains brightly painted pipes, cranks and other mechanisms. At two, my son was thrilled to just look at the "'chines." Unfortunately, the earth is still contaminated. A sign warns against eating the grass, and instructs park users to wash hands after touching the grass, so I don't recommend this park for children who are not yet walking.

★★★★

GREEN LAKE PARK   Wading pool hotline (206)684-7796

7201 E Green Lake Drive, Green Lake

Access: Parking at parking lots around the lake; stroller access
Features: Play equipment for tots (swings, slide, spinner, climbers and other equipment), woodchip and sand play area surfaces, wading pool, restrooms, changing table in community center, some nursing privacy, some shade (no shade over playground)

Green Lake Park is one of the most popular destinations in Seattle. A rebuilt, three-mile long pathway that circles the lake provides wonderful exercise for walkers, runners, skaters and strollers. All around the lake are areas for picnicking and sunbathing. A large wading pool on the north side of the lake teems with children in the summertime. Soccer, softball and volleyball games fill up the playfield on the northeast corner. Sunbathers spread their blankets out everywhere else. On weekends there are often kayak and racing shell competitions.

During weekends and evenings the park is crowded, but the path is large enough for everyone. The popular new playground by the community center has the standard equipment along with some unique pull toys that older toddlers find exciting. Unfortunately, this playground is always crowded and can be overwhelming for small children.

See the Green Lake Community Center description, pages 55-56.

★ ½
MERIDIAN PARK

50th Street and Meridian Avenue NE, Green Lake

Access: Parking; stroller access
Features: Play equipment for tots (swings, slide, climbers), sand play area surface, restrooms, nursing privacy, some shade

No changing table, no food or drink available

Enclosed in a fortress-like wall are the Good Shepherd Center and Meridian Park, a large grassy playsite. The playground has recently been renovated and there are now acceptable apparatuses for younger children. I don't advise going during school hours because a grade school uses this park during recess.

★★ ½
RAVENNA PARK   Wading pool hotline (206)684-7796

Ravenna Boulevard and 21st Avenue NE, Ravenna

Access: Parking; no stroller access
Features: Play equipment for tots (slides, swings, climbers), sand play area surface, wading pool, restrooms, nursing privacy, shade

No changing table, no food or drink available

Ravenna Park is larger than it looks at first glance. The playground is small, but just up a path the park curves toward the west and provides a secluded area with picnic benches and a quiet grassy knoll to lie on and relax. The wading pool is little but warms up quickly in the sun. Oddly, it is located up from the playground, in front of the tennis courts. Despite the playground's diminutive size, it is a very popular place all year long.

★★★½
WALLINGFORD PARK

Wading pool hotline (206)684–7796

43rd Street and Woodlawn Avenue NE, Wallingford

Access: Parking; stroller access

Features: Play equipment for tots (slides, swings, climbers, spinner), sand play area surface, wading pool, restrooms (closed in winter), some shade

No changing table, no food or drink available, no nursing privacy

This park in the Wallingford district is both entertaining and popular. The playground is located next to a large meadow that is ideal for picnics or just lying around. Seven slides, as well as tot swings, regular swings and a tire, provide amusement for youngsters of all ages. The wading pool is not shaded or near grass. I brought my baby here before he could crawl and again after he could walk. He enjoyed himself both times. Wallingford Center is a short walk northeast on 45th Avenue. There you can shop for food, drink, clothes and games for yourself and your baby.

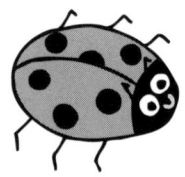

Haller Lake, Northgate, Bitter Lake & Lake City

★★★★
BITTER LAKE PARK Wading pool hotline (206)684–7796

Linden Avenue and 130th Avenue N, Bitter Lake

Access: Parking; stroller access

Features: Play equipment for tots (slides, swings, bouncer, spinner), woodchip play area surface, wading pool, restrooms, changing table in community center, food and drink in community center vending machines and on Aurora Avenue, shade

No nursing privacy

A recently-renovated playground on the southeast corner of Bitter Lake Park sports climbers for all skill levels, bouncers, swings and a wading pool. A sandbox of sorts is available for digging when your little one wants to take a break from running around. A paved pathway parallels the Bitter Lake shore a safe distance from the water. The great numbers of ducks and geese that have found this lake will make it interesting for your little one. Rainy weather leaves grass by the lake soggy.

See the Bitter Lake Community Center description, pages 50-51.

★★
DAHL PLAYGROUND

Wading pool hotline
(206)684–7796

80th Street and 25th Avenue NE, Lake City

Access: Parking; stroller access

Features: Play equipment for tots (slides, swings, climbers, spinner), sand play area surface, wading pool, restrooms, minimal shade

No changing table, no food or drink available, no nursing privacy

Dahl Playground borders busy 25th Avenue, so the park is noisy. However, since it is above the street it is a bit removed from traffic. Interesting play equipment and a wading pool are not well shaded. This is a park for walkers who do not mind lathering up with sunscreen.

★★½
LAKE CITY PARK

123rd Street and 26th Avenue NE, Lake City

Access: Parking; stroller access

Features: Play equipment for tots (slides, bouncer, climbers, spinner), sand play area surface, some nursing privacy, some shade

No restrooms, no changing table, no food or drink available

Play equipment is available to keep baby busy in this quaint park. Paved pathways that meander around the sheared lawn give a feeling of a city park within a residential area. The equipment is old but still in good shape. The major downside to this park is the lack of shade and restrooms.

★★★
LICHTON SPRINGS PARK

97th Street and Ashworth Avenue NE, Northgate

Access: Parking; stroller access

Features: Play equipment for tots (slides, swings, climbers) woodchip play area surface, restrooms, food and drink at Oak Tree Village (six blocks away), some nursing privacy, some shade

No changing table

This historic park is built around Lichton Springs, which were discovered in 1870. The city of Seattle acquired the site in 1960. On the northwest side of the park is a new playground with colorful climbers and other apparatus to play on. The play-lot is not shaded, but you can find shade nearby. A partially paved walkway leads through the park and down to the springs. A quick drive will take you to Oak Tree Village where Larry's Market is one of the places you will be able to find something to eat.

★★
MAPLE LEAF PARK

83rd Street and Roosevelt Way NE, Lake City

Access: Parking; stroller access

Features: Play equipment for tots (slides, swings, climbers, spinner, bouncer), sand play area surface, restrooms out of order when visited

No changing table, no food or drink available, no nursing privacy, no shade

Although there is no shade and the play-lot is just above Roosevelt Way, this is a very popular park. The playground sits between the reservoir to the east and a busy street to the west. A small field next to the lot is also unshaded.

★★½

MATTHEWS BEACH

93rd Street and Sand Point Way NE, North Seattle

Access: Parking; no stroller access
Features: Play equipment for tots (slides, swings, climbers), sand play area surface, restrooms, nursing privacy, shade

No changing table, no food or drink available

Matthews Beach, which lies on the shore of Lake Washington, is both a large park and a beach. The beach is a sliver of sand, so most sunbathing is done on the grass. The playground looks impressive, but may be too challenging for younger toddlers. There are two ways to get to this park. The hard, but fun way is to ride your bike up the Burke-Gilman Trail, with your child in a carrier, until you reach the beach turn off. The easier way is to drive and leave your car in the spacious parking lot.

★★

NORTH ACRES PARK

Wading pool hotline
(206)684–7796

130th Street and 1st Avenue NE, Haller Lake

Access: Parking; stroller access
Features: Play equipment for tots (slides, swings climbers), sand play area surface, wading pool, nursing privacy, shade

No restrooms, no changing table, no food or drink available

This shady park has ample grass and woods as well as a playground with a large sandbox and wading pool. The park also has dirt trails for a jogging stroller or backpack hike, but is dark and a bit rundown. Since it is well shaded, the sand tends to stay wet. The steady hum of traffic resonates from the I–5 freeway located behind the park.

★★★
RICHMOND BEACH

190th Street and 20th Avenue NW, Shoreline

Access: Parking; stroller access up to the sand
Features: Play equipment for tots (slides, swings, climbers), sand play area surface, restrooms, nursing privacy

No changing table, no food or drink available, no shade

At Richmond Beach the parking area is above the beach, and the playground is above the parking lot. A paved path to the beach leads over train tracks to the Sound. However, once at the beach, it is impossible to push your stroller on the sand. The covered picnic area is the only place where you will find shade. This is a fine beach for sunbathing, playing in the sand or swimming in the cold water of Puget Sound.

★★
SACAJAWEA PLAYGROUND

94th Street and 15th Avenue NE, Lake City

Access: Parking; no stroller access
Features: Play equipment for tots (slides, tire, swings, climbers) sand play area surface, nursing privacy, shade

No restrooms, no changing table, no food or drink available

This playground built into a hillside is easy to miss. When driving on NE 94th Street you will first see a field. Just to the west of this field is the play area. A grade school to the north is not near enough to cause any distractions to park visitors. If you live in the area, you will want to visit this park.

★★

VICTORY HEIGHTS PLAYGROUND

105th Street and 19th Avenue NE, Lake City

Access: Parking; stroller access
Features: Play equipment for tots (slides, swings, climbers, spinner) pebble play area surface, restrooms, little shade

No changing table, no food or drink available, no nursing privacy

A small preschool next to this neighborhood park could cause competition for the equipment if the school children are out playing. Other than that, this adequate playground and park may be suitable for you and your baby.

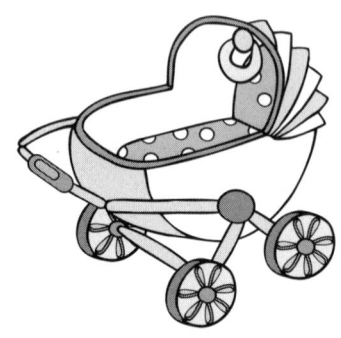

Laurelhurst & View Ridge

★★★½
LAURELHURST PLAYGROUND

41st Street and 46th Avenue NE, Laurelhurst

Access: Parking; stroller access

Features: Play equipment for tots (slides, swings, climbers, spinner), sand play area surface, restrooms, nursing privacy, partial shade

No changing table, no food or drink available

This excellent neighborhood park provides plenty of activity for toddlers. The playground has a variety of equipment for a whole range of ages. There also are open fields for romping or just relaxing. The community center is small, but has a restroom in the basement. Some of the grass and a little of the playground are shaded so your infant can be protected from the sun while your toddler plays on the apparatus.

See the Laurelhurst Community Center description, pages 56–57.

★★★
BRYANT PARK

65th Street and 40th Avenue NE, View Ridge

Access: Parking; stroller access

Features: Play equipment for tots (slides, swings, climbers, spinner, bouncer), woodchip play area surface, food and drink at Puget Consumers Co-op on 65th Street, nursing privacy, some shade

No restrooms, no changing table

This refurbished playground has fresh wood shavings on the play surface instead of dirty sand. Two pieces of climbing equipment have slides; one is appropriate for toddlers. Puget

Consumers Co-op market is right across the street so it's easy to get lunch at their deli or pick up some last-minute items for dinner.

★★★
BURKE-GILMAN PLACE PARK

5200 NE Sandpoint Way, Laurelhurst

Access: Parking; stroller access
Features: Play equipment for tots (slides, swings, climbers), woodchip play area surface, restrooms

No changing table, no food or drink available, no nursing privacy, no shade

Located off the Burke-Gilman Trail, this playground offers a pleasant break to a bicycling parent whose toddler has been riding in a bike trailer for awhile. The playground, rebuilt in the spring of 1999, offers the standard equipment for burning off energy. It is next to a daycare so expect to share the grounds with a group of youngsters on sunny weekdays.

★★★
BURKE-GILMAN TRAIL

Main Access Points: Gas Works Park, Ravenna Boulevard and 25th Avenue NE, Matthews Beach, Tracy Owen Station

Access: Parking; stroller access
Features: Play equipment for tots (see Burke-Gilman Place Park and Matthews Beach), restrooms, shade along the trail

No changing table, no food or drink available, no nursing privacy

The Burke-Gilman Trail was a railroad right-of-way bordering Lake Union and Lake Washington between Gas Works Park and Tracy Owen Station in Kenmore. In 1978 the original 12.1

miles of track were paved over to make a wonderful bike, stroller and walking path. As additional right-of-way has been acquired, the has been extended, and it now starts in Ballard. At Redmond's Blyth Park the Burke-Gilman Trail becomes the Sammamish River Trail, which leads into Marymoor Park in Redmond. I have used a child trailer attached to my bike to take my baby on a smooth ride. If you start at Gas Works Park you will travel over twenty miles to Marymoor Park. There are access points along the path. Burke-Gilman Place Park and Matthews Beach are both accessible from the trail and provide your toddler respite from sitting in a bike trailer.

★★
MAGNUSON PARK   Wading pool hotline (206)684-7796

65th Street and Sandpoint Way NE, View Ridge

Access: Parking; stroller access

Features: Play equipment for tots (slides, swings, climbers, bouncers), woodchip play area surface, wading pool, restrooms, nursing privacy, some shade

No changing table, no food or drink available

In the spring of 1999 the Junior League of Seattle built a large playground at the north end of Magnuson Park. This playground, filled with colorful climbers, is most easily reached via the Naval Station Puget Sound. Don't be intimidated by the manned booth; just tell the officer you want to go to the playground and he will direct you. The waterfront offers swimming in Lake Washington and a large grassy field provides a place for kite flying. There is also an off-leash area for your dog.

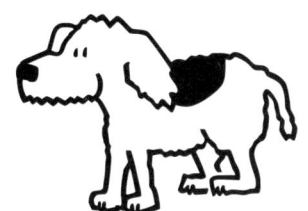

★★½

VIEW RIDGE PARK
Wading pool hotline (206)684-7796

70th Street and 45th Avenue NE, View Ridge

Access: Parking on 45th Avenue; stroller access
Features: Play equipment for tots (slides, swings, climbers, spinner), sand play area surface, wading pool, restrooms, some shade

No changing table, no food or drink available, no nursing privacy

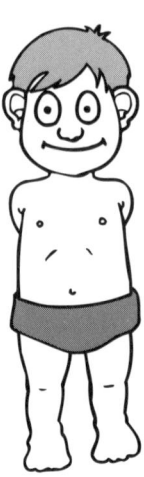

Two separate playgrounds fifty yards apart make up this park. The restrooms and wading pool are in the middle and a large playfield borders both playgrounds on the north. Head for the tot playground on the southwest corner. Unfortunately, parking is available only on 45th Avenue on the east side of the park. Although 70th Street is a large street it is not too noisy.

Ballard, Fremont & Phinney Ridge

★★
BALLARD COMMUNITY CENTER PLAYGROUND

6020 NW 28th Avenue, Ballard

Access: Parking; stroller access
Features: Play equipment for tots (slides, swings, climbers, spinner), sand play area surface, restrooms, food and drink in vending machines, some shade

No changing table, no nursing privacy

This small playground by the Ballard Community Center has a nautical theme. Easily negotiated climbers and slides located on sand are fun for youngsters. Restrooms and vending machines are in the center.

See the Ballard Community Center description, page 48.

★★½
CARKEEK PARK

110th Street and Carkeek Park Road NW, Ballard

Access: Parking; no stroller access
Features: Play equipment for tots (slides, bouncers), pebble play area surface, restrooms, nursing privacy, some shade

No changing table, no food or drink available

This large preserve on Puget Sound has a spectacular view of the Olympic Mountains. To get to the beach, which is below the parking lot, you must walk down a large flight of steps, so the park is not stroller accessible. The creative design of the newly-built playground imitates a fish stream, and has a large salmon-shaped tube slide. Unfortunately, the

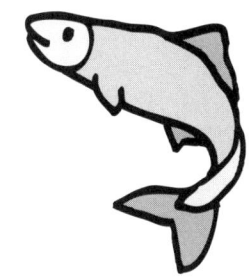

slide is difficult for a small toddler to navigate so I cannot recommend it for unstable walkers. Hiking trails are plentiful; put your baby in a backpack and take a walk.

★★
GILMAN PARK
Wading pool hotline (206)684–7796

54th Street and 11th Avenue NW, Ballard

Access: Parking; stroller access
Features: Play equipment for tots (slides, swings, spinner, low basketball hoop), sand play area surface, wading pool, restrooms, shade

No changing table, no food or drink available, no nursing privacy

This neighborhood park is crowded with older kids on weekends, but is quiet during the week. The shaded wading pool is perfect for hot summer days. The park is near an industrial area to the west, but it doesn't affect the park's atmosphere.

★★★
GOLDEN GARDENS PARK

80th Street and Seaview Avenue NW, Ballard

Access: Parking; stroller access
Features: Play equipment for tots (slides, swings, climbers), sand play area surface, restrooms, food and drink in summer, nursing privacy, some shade

No changing table

Founded in 1929, historic Golden Gardens Park boasts a small playground and a meandering nature walk. The beach affords a beautiful view of the Olympic Mountains. Your little one will enjoy romping on a soft grassy meadow or playing in a shallow creek. The sandy beach provides swimming in cold Puget Sound waters.

★★★½
ROSS PARK

43rd Street and 3rd Avenue NW, Fremont

Access: Parking; stroller access
Features: Play equipment for tots (slides, swings, climbers, spinner), sand play area surface, restrooms, food and drink in mini-market across street, little nursing privacy, some shade

No changing table

Ross Park is my favorite playground in Ballard. Although it doesn't look like much because of its older play equipment, it provides everything needed for a toddler's fun time. Plenty of shade covers one sandy portion of the playground. There is a restroom and picnic bench. A mini-market across the street is convenient for snacks and drinks.

★★★
WEBSTER PARK

3100 NW 68th Street, Ballard

Access: Parking; stroller access
Features: Play equipment for tots (slides, swings, climbers), sand play area surface, portable outhouse

No changing table, no food or drink available, no nursing privacy, no shade

Popular Webster Park is located in front of Ballard's Nordic Heritage Museum. Toddlers and babies abound on the colorful climbers during the morning hours. Next to the playground is a large paved area with a basketball court. This can be used for rolling or running toys. Unfortunately, the only restroom is a portable outhouse. However, that does not seem to deter many neighborhood mothers from visiting this playground.

★★★½

WOODLAND PARK PLAYGROUND

Phinney Ridge and 59th Street N, Phinney Ridge

Access: Parking on street, not in zoo lot; stroller access
Features: Play equipment for tots (slides, swings, climbers, bouncer), sand play area surface, food and drink at 7/11 on Phinney Avenue, some nursing privacy, some shade, but none over playground

No restrooms, no changing table

After opening in June of 1997, this new playground at Woodland Park quickly became very popular. One piece of climbing equipment is especially tot friendly, since it is low to the ground and has wide slides. The park is on the north end of the zoo and is worth a special visit. If your baby does well in a restaurant, go to the Santa Fe Café next to the 7/11. The food is great and the atmosphere is surprisingly child friendly. After ten minutes in any restaurant, my toddler is ready to move on. At the Santa Fe Café my husband can take my toddler to the playground while I have a calm dinner.

★★★★

WOODLAND PARK ZOO   (206)684-4800

601 N 59th Street, Phinney Ridge

Hours: Open daily; summers 9:30 a.m.–6 p.m., winters 9:30 a.m.–4 p.m.;
Fees: Adults 18–64–$8.50; youth 6–17 and disabled–$6.00; preschool 3–5–$3.75; 2 and under–free; seniors 65+–$7.75, annual pass $55; ask for King County residence discount)
Access: Parking in lot ($3.50); stroller access except in the "Night and Day" and "Rainforest" exhibits

Features: Play equipment for tots (slides, climbers, in the center of the zoo grounds), dirt play area surface, restrooms, changing tables in most restrooms, food and drink in large food court, nursing privacy on patches of grass in remote areas, shade

I have always had reservations about zoos. In fact, I thought that I would never take my child to a zoo to see caged animals. Woodland Park Zoo is not that kind of facility. Here the animals are kept in large open habitats quite like their natural environments. Sometimes this hinders viewing, since the animals have a wide area to roam, but it presents a more humane atmosphere to a child. Both paved and unpaved paths meander throughout the zoo giving visitors exceptional peeks into the lives of the various animals. A farm area with a petting zoo offers children a chance to touch tame animals such as goats and sheep. Near the family farm is a play area with things for children to play on and climb over. A large indoor food court displays different types of fare. I took my baby to the zoo as young as five months old and he seemed to get something from the visit. As he gets older he enjoys the experience more and more.

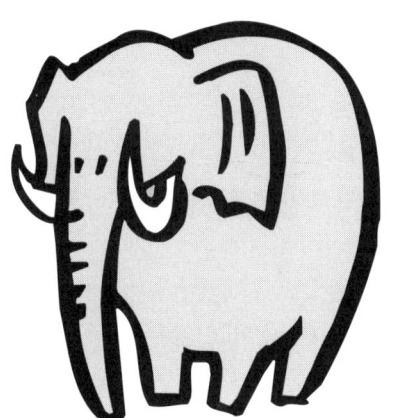

Crown Hill & Loyal Heights

★★★

LOYAL HEIGHTS PLAYGROUND

2101 NW 77th Street, Loyal Heights

Access: Parking; stroller access
Features: Play equipment for tots (slides, swings, climbers, bouncers), woodchip play area surface, restrooms, changing table

No food or drink available, no nursing privacy, no shade

This new tot-lot sports colorful and creative equipment. Bring plenty of sunscreen because there is not much shade. Inside the community center you will find restrooms and indoor activities.

See the Loyal Heights Community Center description, pages 58–59.

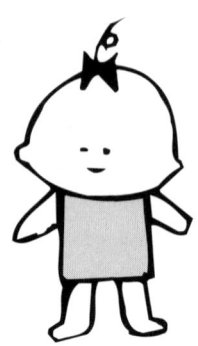

★★½

SALMON BAY PARK

Sloop Place and 19th Avenue NW, Loyal Heights

Access: Parking; stroller access
Features: Play equipment for tots (slides, swings, climbers, spinner, bouncer), sand play area surface, restrooms, shade

No changing table, no food or drink available, no nursing privacy

The recently updated equipment at Salmon Bay Park is bright and colorful. A paved pathway that cuts through rolling woods provides stroller access to the playground at the southeast corner. The restroom is a good distance from the playground, which is inconvenient.

Outdoor Activities & Beaches • Crown Hill & Loyal Heights

★
SANDEL PLAYGROUND

Wading pool hotline
(206)684-7796

92nd Street and 1st Avenue NW, Crown Hill

Access: Parking; stroller access

Features: Play equipment for tots (slides, swings, climbers), sand play area surface, wading pool, restrooms, some nursing privacy, some shade

No changing table, no food or drink available

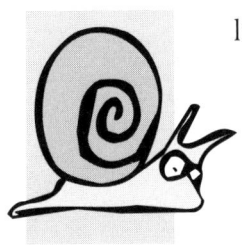

This small playground reminds me of a little cove surrounded by grass and trees. Since the park is below an incline, you cannot see the street from the playground. A pathway loops around the large playfield next to the site.

Shoreline

★½

PARAMOUNT PARK

152nd Street and 10th Avenue NE

Access: Parking; stroller access
Features: Play equipment for tots (slides, climbers), woodchip play area surface

No restrooms, no changing table, no food or drink available, no nursing privacy, no shade

Paramount Park is ideal for joggers who need a smooth track to run with a jog stroller. A paved walkway about the half the length of a football field loops around a large field and playground. There is no shade, so take plenty of sunscreen. The play-lot is not suitable for babies since it lacks a sandbox and tot swing.

★

TWIN PONDS PARK

155th Street and 1st Avenue NE

Access: Parking; stroller access
Features: Play equipment for tots (slides, climbers), pebble play area surface, restrooms (stalls have no doors), some nursing privacy, some shade

No changing table, no food or drink available

The park is located next to the noisy I–5 freeway. A playground and large playfield are near the pond. When I was there it seemed most heavily used by people stopping to use the restroom.

Mercer Island, South Seattle & West Seattle

You'll discover many terrific things to do and places to go in these areas. Rainier Valley parks are found in South Seattle, and both Mercer Island and South Seattle have parks on Lake Washington. West Seattle is full of attractive parks and beaches, many of them on Puget Sound.

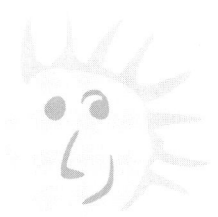

Indoor Activities

ARENA SPORTS   (206)782-8606
4636 E Marginal Way S, #3, Georgetown

Hours and fees: Call for class times and fees
Access: Park in the rear; stroller access
Weekend/evening hours: Yes
Classes: Soccer classes for children three years old and up

Features: Restrooms, changing table, food and drink available, privacy for nursing

Arena Sports does not offer any classes for children under three. Because of this I did not rate them; however, I mention them because they have a playroom where you can take your baby while your older child takes a soccer class. The playroom is filled with toys perfect for toddlers and babies, so the little one is easily entertained. A changing table and private area for nursing is available as well. Park in the rear and use the north entrance if you have a stroller. If the playroom is locked, ask and someone will open it for you.

COOPERATIVE PRESCHOOLS

See Multiple Locations, pages 23–24.

★★★½

DELRIDGE COMMUNITY CENTER   (206)684-7423
4501 SW Delridge Way, West Seattle

Hours and fees: Monday–Friday 10 a.m.–10 p.m. and Saturday 1–8 p.m.; call for class times and fees
Classes: Toddler Mini Gym (under 5 years)
Access: Parking; stroller access
Features: Play equipment for tots (see playground, page 103–104), restrooms, changing table, food and drink in vending machines

No nursing privacy

This is the best open gym that I have investigated. A multitude of balls and toys for riding, pushing and climbing are provided for young toddlers. An Exersaucer and play-gym are available for young infants. Although many children were in the gym when I visited, there were ample toys to go around. The hardwood gym floor makes it easy for tots to play with wheeled toys.

★★★★

LITTLE GYM   (206)524-2623
4636 E Marginal Way S, #3, Georgetown
Other locations: 7777 NE 15th Avenue, Lake City (206)5240--2623; 1800 NE 130th Avenue, Bellevue (425)885-3F866

Hours and fees: Call for class times and fees

Classes: Beasts (1½–2½ years); Super Beasts (2½–3 years)
Access: Parking in the rear; stroller access
Weekend/evening hours: Yes
Features: Play equipment for tots (see below), restrooms, changing table, food and drink available, privacy for nursing

Located in Arena Sports south of Safeco Stadium, this Little Gym offers toddlers and infants a chance to run and crawl as well as bounce on pieces of colorful equipment. At the beginning of the class the instructor sings a welcome song as parents and babies sing and dance in a circle. Free time comes next, giving children an opportunity to explore the equipment. The teacher guides the participants in the best ways to use the equipment to promote the baby's development. After free play everyone gathers for more singing around the large multicolored parachute spread on the floor. Ball playing and then bubble blowing follow the parachute activity. The class ends with a goodbye song. If you have older children, they can take a soccer class at Arena Sports while you and your toddler have fun here.

★★★
MERCER ISLAND BOYS AND GIRLS CLUB   (206)232–4548

2825 W. Mercer Way, Mercer Island

Hours and fees: Call for times and fees
Classes: Open Gym/Rainy Day Playground (under 5 years); open October–June
Access: Parking, no stroller access
Features: Play equipment for tots (see below), restrooms, changing table, drink in vending machines

No nursing privacy, no food

This large gym is filled with trikes, balls, small slides and tumbling cushions, all perfect for the loads of toddlers that come to play. On cool days the gym can be chilly so bring a sweater. The gym floor is wood so your child can speed around on the tricycles and there is enough room so they do not run into the other children. Unfortunately, this gym is open only nine months of the year.

★★
RAINIER FAMILY SUPPORT CENTER (206)723-8590

Rainier Community Center, 4600 S 38th Avenue, South Seattle

Hours and fees: Monday–Thursday 10 a.m.–8 p.m., Friday and Saturday 10 a.m.–5 p.m.; call for class times and fees
Classes: Playroom (age open)
Access: Parking, stroller access
Features: Play equipment for tots (see below), restrooms, changing table, food and drink in vending machines

No nursing privacy

Rainier Family Support Center is located at the entry of the Rainier Community Center. A playroom with toys, blocks and craft supplies is offered free to the public. Call for availability times.

SEATTLE PUBLIC LIBRARIES: TODDLER STORYTIME

Southwest Branch, Holly Park Branch, West Seattle Branch, see Multiple Locations, pages 26–27.

★★★★
SOUTHWEST FAMILY CENTER (206)937-7680

4555 SW Delridge Way, West Seattle

Hours and fees: Monday–Friday 9 a.m.–7 p.m.; call for class times
Classes: PEPS Parent/Child Activity Time (under 3 years); Playroom (all ages)
Access: Parking, stroller access
Features: Play equipment for tots (see below), restrooms, changing table, nursing privacy

No food or drink available

The Southwest Family Center has the best playroom in King County. Not only is it filled with toys for all ages, it is also equipped with a kitchen, diaper changing area, television and VCR. Natural light brightens this large, clean room. Couches and chairs provide spots for parents to relax and read the numerous parenting books provided with their children within easy reach. In the mornings, the room is not busy; in the afternoons it serves as a childcare facility for the center's various classes participants.

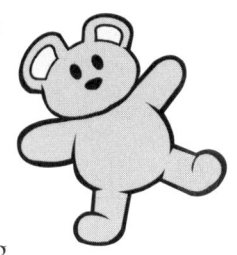

Parent/Child Activity Time. This two-hour activity group is open to parents with children under three years old, although exceptions are made for siblings. The group begins with playtime while the facilitator leads an informal discussion with the parents. Snacks, crafts and singing are also a part of the program.

★★★★
SPECTRUM DANCE THEATER   (206)325-4161

800 Lake Washington Boulevard, Madrona
Classes: Movement with Your Toddler (walking–3 years)
Access: Parking, stroller access
Features: Restrooms

No play equipment for tots, no changing table, no food or drink available, no nursing privacy

Located on Lake Washington, this dance school is co-sponsored by the Seattle Department of Parks and Recreation. The toddler dance class invites children and their parents to join in play exercises. On nice days you can enjoy the sandy beach located below the building.

SWIMMING POOLS: TOT SWIM

Medgar Evers Pool, Mounger Pool, Queen Anne Aquatic Center, Safe 'N Sound Swimming; see Multiple Locations, pages 29–31.

Outdoor Activities & Beaches

MERCER ISLAND

★★
I-90 "LID" PARK

23rd Avenue and Atlantic Street S, Mercer Island

Access: Parking; stroller access
Features: Play equipment for tots (slides, climbers, bouncers), woodchip play area surface, restrooms, nursing privacy

No changing table, no food or drink available, no shade

This large park with plenty of open space and a small sunny playground lies atop the I-90 freeway. The playground and parking lot are located close to the freeway ramps, which makes it convenient for people not living on Mercer Island, but I didn't find much that was outstanding enough to warrant driving here from any distance.

★★
ISLAND CREST PARK

58th Street and Island Crest Way SE

Access: Parking; stroller access
Features: Play equipment for tots (slides, swings, climbers), woodchip play area surface, restrooms, nursing privacy, shade

No changing table, no food or drink available

The playground at Island Crest Park is in a wooded cove located on the north side of this large park. Hiking trails are available for backpackers. A large portion of the grounds is allocated to playfields.

★★★
LUTHER BURBANK PARK

2040 SE 84th Avenue, Mercer Island
Play equipment for tots (slides, swings, climbers), pebble play area surface, restrooms, food and drink in vending machine, nursing privacy, some shade, but none over playground

No changing table

This expansive Mercer Island park sits on the shores of Lake Washington. Walking trails interweave the meadows and restoration projects for easy hikes. The playground is an extensive web of climbing structures and slides that may be too daunting for crawlers or new walkers. Some of the apparatuses are quite high, so it may be difficult for you to sit and watch your toddler make this park a hands-on play experience. The beach lies below the park. Plenty of shade and grass are provided for picnicking and relaxing.

Mount Baker, Rainier Valley & Madrona

★★½
BRIGHTON PLAYGROUND

Juneau Street and 39th Avenue S, Rainier Valley

Access: Parking; some stroller access
Features: Play equipment for tots (slides, swings, climbers, spinner), sand play area surface, restrooms, nursing privacy, shade

No changing table, no food or drink available

This large park stretches over five city blocks. The southwest corner hosts an adequate playground that will entertain your toddler. The climbers are a little advanced so you will have to stand near to give your tot a hand. A playfield is probably used by the high school that borders the park on the south side.

★★½
DEARBORN PARK

Brandon Street and 29th Avenue S, Rainier Valley

Access: Parking minimal; stroller access
Features: Play equipment for tots (slides, swings, climbers), woodchip play area surface, nursing privacy, shade

No restrooms, no changing table, no food or drink available

Located above the street, this small playground is quiet and peaceful. Trees provide plenty of shade on sunny days.

★
MADRONA PARK

900 East Lake Washington Boulevard, Madrona

Access: No parking; stroller access
Features: Restrooms, nursing privacy, shade

No play equipment for tots, no changing table, no food or drink available

This lakefront park affords a beautiful view of Lake Washington and Mercer Island. A beach and a walkway provide a pleasant area to take a stroller. Younger infants may enjoy the beach while crawlers can play on the lush grass. However, keep a close eye as toddlers may find busy Lake Washington Boulevard, which borders the park, a dangerous attraction.

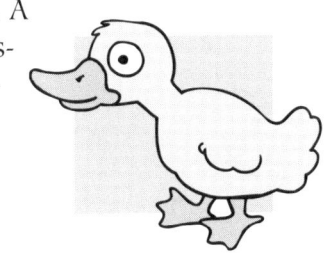

★★½
MOUNT BAKER PARK

Lake Washington Boulevard and Lake Park Drive S, Mount Baker

Access: Parking by lake; stroller access
Features: Play equipment for tots (slides, swings, climbers, bouncers), sand play area surface, restrooms, a little shade

No changing table, no food or drink available, no nursing privacy

Mount Baker Park begins by the lake and continues upward along Lake Park Drive to McClellan Avenue. Parking is available by the beach where there are grassy areas and a nice view of Mercer Island. Get your stroller out and take the wooded path up to the highest part of the park. After walking past a pretty Japanese garden you will come to a large playground. On the sunny Saturday I visited it was full of children.

★★★
OTHELLO PLAYGROUND

Othello Street and 45th Avenue S, Rainier Valley

Access: Parking; stroller access
Features: Play equipment for tots (slides, swings, climbers), pebble play area surface, restrooms, nursing privacy, shade

No changing table, no food or drink available

Beautiful old trees shade quiet areas of this park. Paved pathways interweave throughout the sloping grassy hills. The playground on the northeast corner is brimming with new climbing equipment appropriate for toddlers. A super-slide for older children on the playground's northwest corner is so long that it resembles an amusement park ride.

★★
PRITCHARD BEACH

Gratten Street and Seward Park Avenue S, Rainier Valley

Access: Parking; stroller access
Features: Restrooms, nursing privacy, shade

No play equipment for tots, no changing table, no food or drink available

A sloping lawn leads to a sliver of sandy beach that drops into the water. The dip into the water is gradual, making it safer for toddlers. Few trees are available to provide shade so use of sunscreen is advised.

★★
RAINIER COMMUNITY CENTER PLAYGROUND

Genesee Street and 39th Avenue S, Rainier Valley

Access: Parking; stroller access
Features: Play equipment for tots (slides, spinner, climbers), sand play area surface, restrooms, food and drink in vending machines

No changing table, no nursing privacy, no shade

This large park with a newer community center, is popular with older children. Unfortunately, the center doesn't sponsor any activities for babies. However, the Rainier Family Support Center, which is located here, offers a tot room. The large grassy field has a paved walkway perfect for strollers. Across the street is a larger meadow that leads to Genesee Park.

★★½
SEWARD PARK

Lake Washington Boulevard South and Orcas Street, Rainier Valley

Access: Parking; stroller access
Features: Play equipment for tots (slides, swings, climbers, bouncers), sand play area surface, restrooms, nursing privacy, shade

No changing table, no food or drink available

This 300-acre peninsula park offers splendid views of Lake Washington. The small tot-lot is as popular as the trails and picnic areas. Much of the area is wooded, and dirt paths wind through the trees. There is considerable activity on sunny days but you can still find areas of quiet. Parking can be tight on a sunny weekend since this is a popular destination.

WEST SEATTLE

★★
ALKI BEACH

Alki Beach Road SW, West Seattle

Access: Parking is tight; stroller access
Features: Restrooms, food and drink, some shade

No play equipment for tots, no changing table, no nursing privacy

Sunset magazine rates this Puget Sound attraction as one of Washington's top ten beaches. Sand, grass and a walkway make up this sunny destination. Eating establishments line the street across from the beach. As the beach heads south along the walkway, it is replaced by a sea wall. This is a windy beach with a northwestern exposure, so bundle up if you are heading there on a day that is not warm and sunny. I visited here on a sunny winter day and froze.

★★½
ALKI PLAYGROUND

Lander Street and 59th Avenue SW

Access: Parking; stroller access
Features: Play equipment for tots (slides, climbers), woodchip play area surface, restrooms

No changing table, no food or drink available, no nursing privacy, no shade

This small play-lot was recently refurbished. The equipment is interesting, but there are no swings. Bring sunscreen because the play-lot is unshaded. Unfortunately, the community center does not offer any activities for toddlers and infants.

Outdoor Activities & Beaches • West Seattle

★★½
CAMP LONG (206)684-7434

5200 SW 35th Avenue

Access: Parking; stroller access, but backpack better
Features: Restrooms, nursing privacy, shade

No play equipment for tots, no changing table, no food or drink available

Camp Long is a recreational getaway situated in the West Seattle Golf Course and Recreational Center. Sixty-eight acres are open for hiking, and overnight cabins are available for a fee. There are no programs for toddlers, although activities such as rock climbing and pond ecology are offered to older children. For a good day of family exploring and hiking, Camp Long is an easy place to reach. Ball playing is prohibited in the large field, so little walkers and crawlers can run and you won't have to worry about stray baseballs.

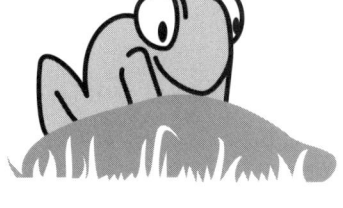

★★
DELRIDGE PARK   Wading pool hotline (206)684-7796

Alaska Street and Delridge Way SW

Access: Parking; stroller access
Features: Play equipment for tots (slides, swings, climbers, spinner), woodchip play area surface, wading pool, restrooms, changing table, food and drink in vending machines, some nursing privacy, some shade

Delridge Park is a small playground located outside the community center, next to a field. Unfortunately, the climbers and slide are difficult for toddlers to use unassisted. The wading pool is a few yards north of the playground. The changing table and vending machines are in the community center. The Delridge Community Center, which offers one of the best open gyms in Seattle, is described on page 92.

★★½

HIAWATHA PLAYGROUND

Wading pool hotline
(206)684–7796

Lander Street and California Avenue SW

Access: Parking; no stroller access
Features: Play equipment for tots (slides, swings, climbers, bouncer), woodchip play area surface, wading pool, restrooms, food and drink nearby at Puget Consumers Co-op and McDonalds, nursing privacy, shade

No changing table

This multi-purpose park has a brand new playground. Tennis courts, playfields and a community center make this a popular destination in West Seattle. The playground is in the middle of a shaded grove which helps keep things cool on hot summer days. The wading pool is a bit far from the playground. Unfortunately, the community center does not offer any activities for children under three.

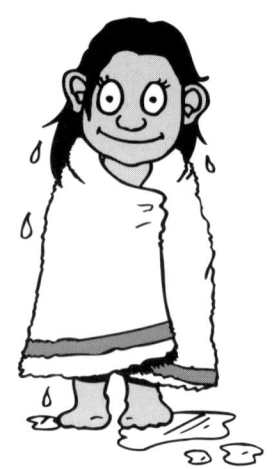

★★
HIGHLAND PARK
Wading pool hotline (206)684-7796

Trenton Street and 11th Avenue SW

Access: Parking; stroller access
Features: Play equipment for tots (swings, climbers) sand play area surface, wading pool, restrooms (closed in winter), minimal shade

No changing table, no food or drink available, no nursing privacy

Highland Park is primarily for older children. However, its two separate playgrounds do have some attractions for toddlers. The first play area is situated in a large playfield. It has a swings and climbers on sand and an unshaded wading pool. The second playground, which is next to the elementary school, has additional equipment with wood shavings underneath.

★
HIGHPOINT PARK

Myrtle Street and 34th Avenue SW

Access: Parking; stroller access
Features: Play equipment for tots (slides, climbers), astroturf play area surface, restrooms, shade

No changing table, no food or drink available, no nursing privacy

Highpoint Park, named because it is at the highest point in West Seattle, provides a view east to the city. A small play area uphill from a large ballfield is nice to visit, although its climbers are too advanced for toddlers. Highpoint Community Center, which stands to the north of the play area, does not have activities for babies. This would be a good place to stop by if an older brother or sister were in a league playing in the field below and you had to wait with your little one.

★★★
LAKEWOOD PARK

110th Street and 10th Avenue SW

Access: Parking; stroller access
Features: Play equipment for tots (slides, swings, climbers), sand play area surface, restrooms, little nursing privacy, shade

No changing table, no food or drink available

This picturesque park wraps around a small lake. A paved pathway leads around the lake and through a meadow. Two separate play areas are available to explore. This is a pretty setting for an afternoon break.

★★★★
LINCOLN PARK   Wading pool hotline (206)684–7796

8400 SW Fauntleroy Way

Access: Parking; jog stroller access
Features: Play equipment for tots (slides, swings, climbers, bouncer), woodchip play area surface, wading pool, restrooms, nursing privacy, shade

No changing table, no food or drink available

This magnificent multi-purpose park, lying on the shores of Puget Sound, hosts many family and group picnics. Dirt trails interweave throughout the woods, making standard strollers difficult to roll. The playground located in the northern portion of the park is actually two separate play areas plus a kidney-shaped wading pool. The first play area contains climbers for children of any age. The other tot-sized area boasts convenient nearby picnic benches. Trees shade many areas of the park, so you can stay out of the sun if you wish. This is a popular destination, so arrive early if you're planning a visit on a sunny weekend.

★
RIVERVIEW PLAYFIELD

Othello Street and 12th Avenue SW

Access: Parking; stroller access
Features: Play equipment for tots (slides, swings, climbers), sand play area surface, restrooms at south end of park, some shade

No changing table, no food or drink available, no nursing privacy

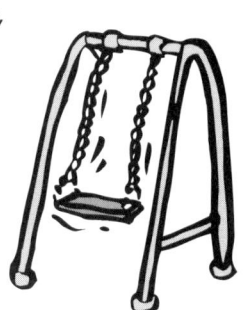

A large two-block playfield leaves space for a small playground in the northern section of this multipurpose park. Little League players use another area north of the playground. Residences lining 12th Avenue make this a quiet street.

★★
SEACREST PARK

1900 SW Seacrest Park

Access: Parking; stroller access
Features: Restrooms, food and drink across the street

No play equipment for tots, no changing table, no nursing privacy, no shade

A paved walkway that runs along the east side of West Seattle, overlooking Elliot Bay, is suitable for all types of strollers. Seacrest Park can be windy because it borders the Sound; however, it is popular spot the entire year. Find food and a spot to eat at restaurants and delis that are across the street, or take the path to a grassy area with picnic tables. Farther north, the path eventually turns into a walkway along the road that borders the sea wall. If you have an active walker you may want to avoid this park because it is so close to the water.

The Eastside

Among the suburbs on the east side of Lake Washington are the popular cities of Bellevue, Medina, Kirkland, Redmond, Issaquah and Renton. Because these rapidly-growing areas boast many families with children you will find a wealth of indoor and outdoor activities for babies.

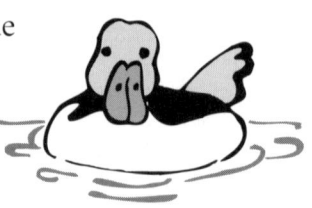

Indoor Activities

★★★

ANDERSON PARK/REDMOND PARKS AND RECREATION (425)556–2300

7802 NE 168th Avenue, Redmond

Hours and fees: Monday–Friday 8 a.m.–5 p.m.; call for class times and fees

Classes: Kindermusik Beginnings (18 months–3 years); Kindermusik Villages (0–17 months); Rainbow Makers (2–3 years); Teenie Weenie Wigglers (2–3 years)

Access: Parking; stroller access

Features: Play equipment for tots (see below), restrooms, food and drink nearby

No changing table, no nursing privacy.

This wooded city park hosts a number of activities in its two cottage-like houses, the Adair House and the Fullard House. A small playground adorns the southeast tip of the park.

Kindermusik Beginnings. Once a week parents and children meet in the Adiar House for a half hour of musical fun.

Children are encouraged to explore music through singing, dancing and playing musical instruments.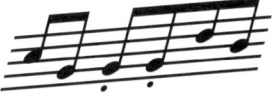

Kindermusik Villages. This class, which is specifically for infants with their parents, introduces young babies to music.

Rainbow Makers. This arts and crafts time, designed for children to create projects with various mediums, meets in the Fullard House for forty-five minutes once a week for eight weeks.

Teenie Weenie Wigglers. Movement, singing and dance are designed to give your child a sense of rhythm and spatial awareness. Parents remain with the children. The class meets in the Fullard House for forty-five minutes once a week.

Redmond Park District also sponsors other seasonal and outdoor classes that meet periodically throughout the year. Call (425)556-2300 for a recreation guide.

See the Anderson Park description, page 132.

BARNES AND NOBLE: STORYTIME

See Multiple Locations, pages 27–28.

★★
BELLEVUE FAMILY YMCA   (425)746-9900

14230 Bel-Red Road, Bellevue

Hours and fees: Monday–Thursday 5 a.m.–10 p.m., Friday 5 a.m.–9 p.m., Saturday and Sunday 8 a.m.–6 p.m.; call for class times and fees
Classes: Parent/Tot Swim (6 months–3 years)
Weekend/evening hours: Yes
Access: Parking; stroller access
Features: Play equipment for tots (see below), restrooms, changing table, food and drink in vending machines
No nursing privacy

At the Bellevue YMCA parents accompany their children in the pool for a thirty-minute-session. Memberships include a one-time joining fee as well as a monthly charge. Non-members can participate in the swim lessons for a small fee. The facility offers other programs for adults and older children, but nothing else for toddlers. For $1 an hour, with a two hour maximum, an on-site nursery provides care for your toddler or infant if you are in an aerobic class.

BORDERS BOOKS: STORYTIME

See Multiple Locations, pages 27–28.

COOPERATIVE PRESCHOOLS

See Multiple Locations, pages 23–24.

★★
CROSSROADS COMMUNITY CENTER   (425)452-4874

1600 NE 10th Street, Bellevue

Hours and fees: Monday–Friday 9 a.m.–8 p.m. and Saturday 9 a.m.–5 p.m.; call for class times and fees
Classes: Playgroup (under 5 years)
Access: Parking; stroller access
Features: Play equipment for tots (see below), restrooms, food and drink in vending machines

No changing table, no nursing privacy

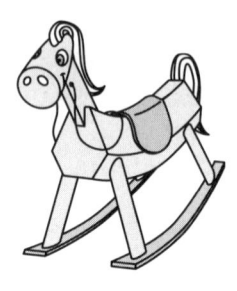

For two hours on Fridays the Crossroads Community Center opens its large gym to parents with children under five. Usually there are fewer than ten children at any one time. The center provides bikes, balls, toys and mats. Parents are required to set up and take down the equipment.

See the Crossroads Playground description, page 125.

Indoor Activities

★★★★
FIRST STEPS (425)392-2095
Gilman Village, 317 NW Gilman Boulevard, #9, Issaquah

Hours and fees: Call for class times and fees
Classes: Smiling, Sitting and Crawling (3–9 months); On the Go (8–14 months); Born to Run (12–24 months); Toddleriffic (16–24 months); Chatter Box (22–30 months); Imagine That (2½–3½years); Mini Michelangelo (18 months and up); Play to Learn Spanish (2 years and up); Discover Science (2 years and up); Free Community Play Time (all ages)
Weekend/evening hours: Yes
Access: Parking; no stroller access
Features: Play equipment for tots, restrooms, changing table, food and drink in nearby restaurants, nursing privacy

The first six classes listed here are similarly organized, but activities vary according to the developmental stage of the participants. Each eight-hour class begins with circle time, in which everyone sings and uses hand motions to a particular theme of the day, such as "fish." After circle time the children can play freely with the toys provided. Then everyone joins together for big circle time where they explore movement and and play finger games. A large parachute is brought out for more fun and learning. Toward the end of class parents participate in a discussion while the children munch on snacks.

Mini-Michelangelo. This art class provides toddlers a chance to use hands, fingers and paintbrushes with paint, playdough and crayons to create their own masterpieces.

Play to Learn Spanish. For 1½ hours parents leave the children to learn Spanish through play, music and other activities.

Discover Science. Toddlers will be encouraged to explore science.

Community PlayTime. Twice a week, First Steps opens up its playroom for drop-in fun. Parents stay with their children.

GYMBOREE

See Multiple Locations, pages 24–25.

★★½
HIGHLAND COMMUNITY CENTER   (425)452-7686

14224 Bel-Red Road, Bellevue

Hours and fees: Monday–Thursday 9 a.m.–8 p.m., Friday and Saturday 9 a.m.–5 p.m.; call for class times and fees
Classes: Open gym (under 5 years)
Weekend/evening hours: Nothing offered for tots
Access: Parking; stroller access
Features: Play equipment for tots (see below), restrooms, food and drink in vending machines

No changing table, no nursing privacy

This community center offers a large gym filled with all sorts of toys for children under five. It's perfect for rainy days— take your toddler here for running, riding and playing with a wide variety of items. The center does not offer any specialized classes for toddlers and infants but this open gym makes up for the loss.

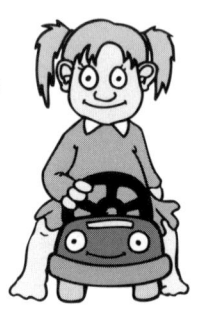

★★★★
ISSAQUAH COMMUNITY CENTER   (425)837-3300

301 S Rainier Boulevard, Issaquah

Hours and fees: Monday, Wednesday, Friday 6 a.m.–10 p.m., Tuesday, Thursday 7 a.m.–10 p.m., Saturday 9 a.m.–4 p.m.; call for class times and fees
Classes: Kids Korner (1–4 years); Toddler Time (1–3 years); Little Gym (19–27 months and 27–36 months)
Weekend/evening hours: Nothing offered for tots

Access: Parking; stroller access
Features: Play equipment for tots (see below), restrooms, changing table, food and drink in vending machines
No nursing privacy

From the outside, the Issaquah Community Center looks more like an expensive health club than a city community center; inside, the facilities are just as nice. Most of the activities are housed in the huge carpeted gym that is divided into three sections.

Kids Korner. A drop-in daycare is available to parents who wish to use the pool or other center facilities. Up to eight children are cared for at one time. Parents who make reservations 48 hours in advance pay a discounted rate.

Toddler Time. Toddlers enjoy one third of the large gym to play with the toys, bikes, slides and many other toys that the center provides. Carpeting makes any falls a little softer.

Little Gym. The Little Gym comes to the center to provide its classes to toddlers up to three years old, as well as older children. This program uses various tumbling equipment to enhance a youngster's coordination, confidence and development.

★★
ISSAQUAH TRAIN DEPOT MUSEUM (425)392-2322

Front Street and Sunset Way, Issaquah

Hours and fees: Saturday 11 a.m.–3 p.m. (free)
Weekend/evening hours: Yes
Access: Parking; stroller access
Features: Restrooms

No play equipment for tots: no changing table, no food or drink available, no nursing privacy

Two sets of railroad tracks straddle this small museum. Located in a replica of a train station, it houses logging train memorabilia, historical facts and artifacts of a time gone by. An old caboose, passenger train and a couple of other industrial trains that sit in front of the museum are available to explore. When the museum is closed, the trains can still be viewed.

★★½

KELSEY CREEK COMMUNITY PARK   (425)452-7688

13204 SE 8th Place, Bellevue

Hours and fees: Daily 9:30 a.m.–4 p.m.; call for class times and fees
Classes: Forty-five minute tour of farm; Clay Expressions (2½–6 years)
Access: Parking; stroller access
Features: Play equipment for tots (playground), restrooms,

No changing table, no food or drink available, no nursing privacy

Clay Expressions. For over an hour, a qualified pottery instructor shows classes of up to six children with their parents how to use clay as an art form, and are encouraged to experiment with clay. This class may move out of Kelsey Creek, so please phone to inquire.

See the Kelsey Creek Park description, page 127.

★★★★

THE LITTLE GYM   (425)885-3866

1800 130th Avenue NE, Bellevue
Other Locations: 7777 15th Avenue NE, Lake City, (206)524–2623; 4636 E Marginal Way S, Georgetown, (206) 524-2623

Hours and fees: Call for times and fees of classes
Classes: Bugs (4–10 months), Birds (10–19 months), Beasts (19 months–2½ years)
Weekend/evening hours: Yes

Indoor Activities

Access: Parking; stroller access
Features: Play equipment for tots (see below), restrooms, changing table

No food or drink available, no nursing privacy

These loosely-structured classes give toddlers and infants a chance to run, crawl, climb and bounce on colorful pieces of equipment. Classes consist of singing and group movement, and also allow free time to explore the equipment. An instructor is on hand to assist parents in teaching their child various methods of using the apparatus. After free play, everyone gathers around the large multicolored parachute for singing and play. The class ends with a good-bye song. These gyms are very stimulating for babies.

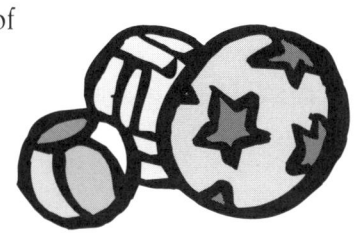

★★★★
MOM'S GROUP   (425)827-3077 Contact: Kathy Smith

St. John's Episcopal Church, 105 State Street, Kirkland

Hours and fees: Call for time of meetings and fees
Classes: Support Group (0–5 years)
Access: Parking; stroller access
Features: Play equipment for tots (see below), restrooms, changing table, nursing privacy

No food or drink available

Although St. John's Episcopal Church sponsors this support group for mothers, you do not have to be a church member to join. Six to eight mothers of children under five meet once a week for an informal discussion of motherhood, parenting and other concerns that arise. Children are cared for at the church's nursery so the meeting is uninterrupted. However, if your baby is going through separation anxiety you are encouraged to keep it with you.

★★★★

MOTHERS AND OTHERS (425)226–6600

St. Madeline Sophie Catholic Church
4400 SE 130th Place, Rooms J, K and L, Bellevue

Hours and fees: Call for time and fee of meetings
Classes: Support group, childcare available
Access: Parking; stroller access
Features: Play equipment for tots (see below), restrooms, changing table, nursing privacy

No food or drink available

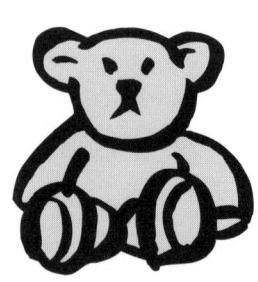

Mothers, fathers and caregivers are welcome to meet two hours weekly for informative discussions, speakers and activities. During the school year between twenty-five to sixty mothers, fathers, grandparents and nannies gather once a week at the church. Children are left with caregivers while the parents meet separately. Infants are tended to in one area, toddlers play together in a separate room and preschoolers experience a more structured class. You may keep your baby with you if necessary. In the summer, the group meets at various parks in the area. The facilitators also organize Mom's Night Out and family events.

★★★★

NORTH KIRKLAND COMMUNITY CENTER (425)828–1105

12421 NE 103rd Avenue, Kirkland

Hours and fees: Monday–Friday 8 a.m.–5 p.m. Open for classes on Saturday; call for class times and fees

Classes: Indoor Playground (1–5 years); Parent/Child Art (2 –3½ years); Parent/Toddler Movement (12–18 months); Parent/Child Movement (18–30 months); Preschool Movement (2½–3 years); Parent/Child Music (2–3½ years)
Weekend/evening hours: Yes
Access: Parking; stroller access
Features: Play equipment for tots (see below), restrooms, changing table, food and drink in vending machines

No nursing privacy

This small community center has a large number of activities for youngsters.

Indoor Playground. Toys and games are available for youngsters. The playground is not opened year-round so be sure to call ahead.

Parent/Child Art. Parents guide their toddlers through various artistic endeavors. Butcher paper is placed on the walls for chalk use. Your child can use finger paints, glue with dry pasta and ink stamps without dirtying your house

Parent/Toddler Movement, Parent/Child Movement and Preschool Movement. In these classes, the tumbling equipment is similar to Gymboree and Little Gym, although the room where it is held is much smaller. An instructor guides you and your child through various exercises, games and songs. During Preschool Movement, the children participate without their parents.

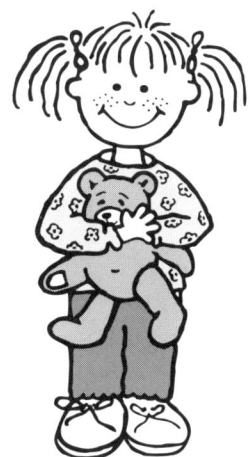

Parent/Child Music. This forty-five minute class introduces your toddler to the basic concepts of music. Parents stay with the toddlers as they experiment with instruments and songs.

See the North Kirkland Park description, page 138

★★★½

NORTHWEST CENTER   (425)452-6046

9825 NE 24th Street, Bellevue

Hours and fees: Monday–Friday 8 a.m.–5 p.m.; call for class times and fees

Classes: Pee Wee Picasso (18 months–2½ years); Kindermusik Beginnings (18 mo.–2½ years); Kindermusik Villages (0–17 months); Romp and Roll (18 months–2½ years); Musical Magic (2–3 years)

Access: Parking; stroller access

Features: Play equipment for tots (see below). restrooms, changing table

No nursing privacy, no food or drink available

This center primarily consists of classrooms, however its diminutive size in no way minimizes the opportunities for children under three.

Pee Wee Picasso. Up to eight toddlers experiment with different crafts. Four low tables are set with different activities for the little ones. The forty-five minute class is led by an instructor who is assisted by parents.

Kindermusik Beginnings. This half-hour class allows toddlers to experience music through singing, listening and creating music. Musical instruments such as bells and rattles are used.

Kindermusik Villages. This Kindermusik class offers a chance to expose the youngest baby to music.

Romp and Roll. For forty-five minutes your tot uses exercise and singing to emphasize coordination, listening and social skills. The class is kept small, with a maximum of ten children, each with a parent.

Musical Magic. Older toddlers with their parents operate rhythm instruments, sing songs and play with finger puppets for forty-five minutes.

Indoor Activities

★★★½
PLAYSPACE AT CROSSROADS MALL (425)644-4500

8th Street and 156th Avenue NE, Bellevue

Hours and fees: Monday–Thursday 10 a.m.–9 p.m., Friday and Saturday 10 a.m.–10:30 p.m., Sunday 11 a.m.–6 p.m., ($4.50 per child); Drop-off Care ($5.50 first hour, additional hours $4), Parents Night Out ($15 first child, $12 additional children)
Access: Parking; stroller access
Features: Play equipment for tots, restrooms, changing table, food and drink in mall

No nursing privacy

Playspace at Crossroads Mall has been recently remodeled. Now, children eight-years-old and under can play on a large tubular structure with ball pits and slides. Blocks, Legos® and other toys are also available. A large-screen television displays video cartoons. Your potty-trained child can be left for up to four hours. This is an excellent place to take more than one child, as there are many things to keep everyone busy.

PUBLIC LIBRARIES: TODDLER STORYTIME

Newport Way Library, Lake Hills Library, Issaquah Library, Bellevue Regional Library, Kirkland Public Library, see Multiple Locations, pages 26–27.

★★★★
RENTON COMMUNITY CENTER (425)235-2560

1715 Maple Valley Highway, Renton

Hours and fees: Hours: Monday–Thursday 9 a.m.–9 p.m., Friday and Saturday 10 a.m.–6 p.m. call for class times and fees

Classes: Kindermusik Village (newborn–18 months); Terrific Tots Playground (10 months–3 years); Messy Time for 2's (2 years); Parent/Infant Class (newborn–6 months); Toddlersize (2–3 years)
Weekend/evening hours: Yes
Access: Parking; stroller access
Features: Play equipment for tots (see below), restrooms, changing table, food and drink in vending machines

No nursing privacy

The City of Renton has provided well in this community center filled with classes for children under three. Although there is no drop-in activity, you can register your newborn, infant or toddler for a number of different offerings. Also, there is a preschool called Almost 3's Preschool that is designed for youngsters who are about to turn three.

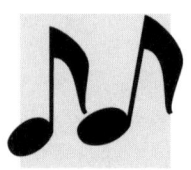

Kindermusik Village. This Kindermusik class provides musical stimulation for newborns, infants and toddlers. The session meets for forty-five minutes once a week.

Terrific Tots Playground. This is an indoor playground that meets three days a week for an hour and a half. You can sign up for one, two or all three days a week. Parents must stay with their child, but the center provides the toys.

Messy Time for 2's. Two year olds can express themselves with various art mediums for forty-five minutes once a week. Parents stay with their children.

Parent/Infant Class. A nurse teaches parents about infant development and more. Parents take their baby to this ninety-minute class.

Toddlersize. For forty-five minutes once a week, toddlers and their parents or nannies can participate in group activities for playing and learning.

★★★½

SAMENA SWIM AND RECREATION CLUB (425)746-1160

15231 Lake Hills Boulevard, Bellevue

Hours and fees: Monday–Friday 5 a.m.–10 p.m., Saturday 7 a.m.–10 p.m., Sunday 9 a.m.–10 p.m. Call for class times and fees and times that childcare is available
Classes: Kindermusik Beginnings (18 months–3½ years); Kindermusik Villages (0–18 months); Childcare (Infants–8 years)
Weekend/evening hours: Nothing for tots available
Access: Parking; stroller access
Features: Play equipment for tots (in play area), restrooms, food and drink

No nursing privacy

This fitness and swim club has been serving the Eastside for forty years. Members enjoy a full range of activities. In addition to swimming and fitness equipment the club offers dance, yoga, aerobic classes and more. Their many classes, including those for infants and toddlers, are open to both members and nonmembers.

Kindermusik Beginnings. Once a week children and their caregivers meet for a half-hour of musical fun. Children are encouraged to explore music through singing, dancing and playing musical instruments.

Kindermusik Villages. This class, which introduces music to young children, is specifically for infants with their parents.

STARS: STORYTIME

See Multiple Locations, pages 27–28.

SWIMMING POOLS: TOT SWIM

Bellevue Aquatics Center, Issaqah's Julius Boehm Pool, Peter Kirk Pool, Redmond City Pool, Bellevue Family YMCA, Water-babies Aquatic Program, see Multiple Locations, pages 29–31.

★★★
VILLAGE THEATRE (425)392–2202

303 Front Street North, Issaquah

Hours and fees: Box office open Tuesday–Saturday 11 a.m.–7 p.m. Call for shows, times and fees
Weekend/evening hours: Yes
Access: Parking; stroller access
Features: Restrooms, food and drink in café next door, nursing privacy

No play equipment for tots, no changing table,

    This Issaquah theatre features live family productions. The theater's two family rooms are strategically located for fine viewing. These soundproof rooms are less expensive than the regular seating. You'll find it's a great way to attend the theater with your infant without worrying about feeding or possible crying.

★★
WEST HILLS FAMILY ENRICHMENT CENTER (206)772–2050

12704 S 76th Avenue South, Renton

Hours and fees: Monday–Friday 9 a.m.–5 p.m.; call for class times and fees
Classes: PEPS–Parent/Child Playtime (under 3 years); Playroom (age open)
Access: Parking; stroller access
Features: Play equipment for tots (see below), restrooms, nursing privacy

No changing table, no food or drink available

    The small playroom at West Hills Family Enrichment Center is available to parents and children during the center's open hours.
    Parent/Child Playtime. On Tuesdays, PEPS sponsors Parent/Child Playtime for preschoolers, toddlers and infants. For two hours on Tuesday afternoons, parents and caregivers meet with a facilitator for music, games, art and playtime.

Outdoor Activities & Beaches

Bellevue & Medina

★★½
ARDMORE PARK

30th Street and 168th Place NE, Bellevue

Access: Parking on street; no stroller access
Features: Play equipment for tots (slides, swings, climbers, bouncers), woodchip play area surface, nursing privacy, shade

No restrooms, no changing table, no food or drink available

At Ardmore Park, a small forest of tall evergreen trees to the south of the playground provides morning shade on sunny days and offers trails for hiking with baby in a backpack. The playground boasts newer play equipment; an open field graces the park's west side

★★★
BOVEE PARK

1500 NE 108th Avenue, Bellevue

Access: Parking; stroller access (gravel path)
Features: Play equipment for tots (slides, swings, climbers, bouncers), woodchip play area surface, restrooms (closed off-season), nursing privacy, shade

No changing table, no food or drink available

A wide gravel path passes by a quiet, shady plat, then leads to a small playground. With plenty of shade and restrooms close by, the spot is perfect for small gatherings of caregivers and their babies. The slides in the playground, which are accessed by rope ladders, could be too difficult for new walkers; however, the bouncers and swings will entertain toddlers of any skill level.

★★½
CITY OF BELLEVUE DOWNTOWN PARK

4th Street and 100th Avenue NE, Bellevue

Access: Parking; stroller access
Features: Play equipment for tots (slides, swings, climbers, bouncers), woodchip play area surface, portable toilets, food and drink within walking distance

No changing table, no nursing privacy, no shade

This colorful, vibrant playground is across the road from Bellevue Square. The play-lot is near a large water fountain and gathering area. A paved walkway traverses a grassy portion of the park. The tot-lot and park are popular throughout the year. At noon, many office workers eat lunch on the park benches. Food can be found on Main Street and at Bellevue Square.

★★
CLYDE BEACH PARK

92nd Street and Lake Washington Boulevard East, Bellevue

Access: Parking; stroller access
Features: Play equipment for tots (slides, climbers), sand play area surface, restrooms

No changing table, no food or drink available, no nursing privacy, no shade

Located on Lake Washington, small Clyde Beach Park is a place where older kids may want to swim. Toddlers will be attracted to the boat-shaped climbing structure. This "boat" is basically the entire playground, but it has enough ins and outs and ups and downs to keep any child busy. There is a field behind the playground, but it is a little too steep for babies to enjoy.

★★★
CROSSROADS PARK

8th Street and 160th Avenue NE, Bellevue

Access: Parking; stroller access
Features: Play equipment for tots (slides, swings, climbers, bouncers), woodchip play area surface, restrooms, food and drink at Crossroads Mall, shade,

No changing table, no nursing privacy

This playground, which is popular with the under-three set, is behind the Crossroads Community Center and next to a large grassy field. A paved pathway meanders through the park. There is ample shade along the grassy parkway. Restrooms and vending machines are in the community center.

See the Crossroads Community Center description, page 110.

★
FOREST HILL PARK

13232 SE 51st Street, Bellevue

Access: Street parking; no stroller access
Features: Play equipment for tots (slides, swings, climbers), astroturf play area surface

No restrooms, no changing table, no food or drink available, no nursing privacy, no shade

A dirt path about the length of a high school track loops around the sunny playground at Forest Hill Park. If your stroller can be managed well over grass, you can reach the playground with it. Since it is a couple of hundred feet from the street, you may prefer to use your stroller regardless of the difficulty. There is no shade so you'll want to keep your visit short on sunny days. This park is best to visit if you live nearby, since parking is scarce.

★★
HILLAIRE PARK

6th Street and 160th Avenue NE, Bellevue

Access: Parking; stroller access
Features: Play equipment for tots (slides, swings, climbers), woodchip play area surface, restrooms, little shade

No changing table, no food or drink available, no nursing privacy

This quiet neighborhood park is located far enough from Crossroads Mall to offer some privacy. Since it is small and unshaded it is probably best to come here in the early morning.

★★½
IVANHOE PARK

Northup Way and 168th Avenue NE, Bellevue

Access: Parking; no stroller access
Features: Play equipment for tots (slides, swings, climbers, bouncers), woodchip play area surface, nursing privacy, shade

No restrooms, no changing table, no food or drink available

Large evergreens shade this little playground and park. On a drizzly spring day the park may seem dark, but on a hot summer day it is an ideal place to take your sun-sensitive baby. You can sit on a blanket of grass under a tree while your toddler enjoys well-shaded play equipment.

★★½
KELSEY CREEK COMMUNITY PARK   (425)455-7688

13204 SE 8th Place, Bellevue

Access: Parking; stroller access
Features: Play equipment for tots (slides, swings, climbers, bouncers), astroturf play area surface, restrooms, food and drink in vending machines, some shade

No changing table, no nursing privacy

Kelsey Creek Park is a huge park with a colorful play area suitable for new walkers. Several grassy areas are available for sitting with younger babies. Hiking trails wind around the park, so take your child carrier to enjoy these.

Kelsey Creek Farm, which is just above the playground, is open to the public and offers children the opportunity to see farm animals up close. The farm has many activities geared toward children three years old and older. A forty-five minute farm tour may be fun for younger toddlers as well as older children.

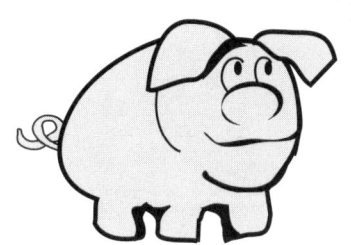

See the Kelsey Creek Farm description, page 114.

★★½
KILLARNEY GLEN PARK

19th Street and 104th Avenue SE, Bellevue

Access: Parking; no stroller access
Features: Play equipment for tots (slides, swings, climbers), woodchip play area surface, nursing privacy, shade

No restrooms, no changing table, no food or drink available

A charming playground, tennis courts and an open field await you in the midst of a evergreen forest at Killarney Glen

Park. Hiking trails weave in and out of the wooded boundary and a sunny meadow provides a superb area for picnics. The absence of a restroom makes a lengthy visit impractical.

★★★★
LAKE HILLS PARK

14th Street and 164th Avenue SE, Bellevue

Access: Parking; stroller access
Features: Play equipment for tots (slides, swings, climbers), woodchip play area surface, restrooms, some shade

No changing table, no food or drink available, no nursing privacy

This four-star park is divided into two sections: One part has an apparatus in the shape of a ship for small children to climb on; the second is filled with all types of pipes, rings and slides for climbing and swinging. A pathway leads to a bridge with slides descending into the play area. Although this equipment was too advanced for my one-year-old, he loved watching the excited play of three-and four-year-olds

★★½
LAKEMONT COMMUNITY PARK

5170 E Village Park Drive, Bellevue

Access: Parking; stroller access
Features: Play equipment for tots (slides, swings, climbers), woodchip play area surface, restrooms: Yes

No changing table, no food or drink available, no nursing privacy, no shade

Large Lakemont Community Park lies north of Village Drive, the road leading into the Lakemont development. Here, tennis courts, trails, basketball courts and a playground are available to the public. The sunny playground sports a boat-shaped play structure that is fun for toddlers, although the slide may be too high for most.

★★★
LAKEMONT HIGHLANDS PARK

15800 SE 63rd Street, Bellevue

Access: Parking; stroller access
Features: Play equipment for tots (slides, swings, climbers), astroturf and woodchip play area surface

No restrooms, no changing table, no food or drink available
no nursing privacy, no shade

This beautifully landscaped playground is built into a small hillside. At the top of the hill are climbers, then slides that resemble a waterfall cascade down. At the bottom of the slides is another playground with swings. If the small parking lot on 63rd Street is full you can park on 62nd Street and take the paved path to the play areas.

★★★
MEYDENBAUER BEACH PARK

419 NE 98th Avenue, Bellevue

Access: Parking; stroller access
Features: Play equipment for tots (slides, swings, climbers, bouncers), pebble play area surface, restrooms, nursing privacy, some shade

No changing table, no food or drink available

At Meydenbauer Beach Park a paved walkway leads you under Lake Washington Boulevard, connecting the parking lot to the beach and playground. It is quite a jaunt and going down is effortless, but be aware that you'll have to push your stroller or carry a tired tot all the way back up to the car. The small, sunny playground has an easy climber; however, the slide is a bit steep. A smidgen of beach on Lake Washington is available for digging in sand or wading; lots of grass fills in the remainder of the park.

★★★

MEDINA PARK

12th Street and 80th Avenue NE, Medina

Access: Parking; jog stroller access
Features: Play equipment for tots (slides, climbers), woodchip play area surface, restrooms, nursing privacy, some shade

No changing table, no food or drink available

Grassy slopes surrounding a quaint duck pond at this beautifully landscaped park. A gravel path loops around the rustic site. The play-lot is small and unshaded but it is adequate for the children playing there. It is a pleasant park to visit with pre-crawlers who are happy sitting still on the lush grass while you take in the scenery.

★

NEWPORT HILLS PARK

60th Street and 120th Avenue SE, Bellevue

Access: Parking; stroller access
Features: Play equipment for tots (swings, climbers), pebble play area surface, restrooms

no changing table, no food or drink available, no nursing privacy, no shade

If you live in the Newport Hills area and want to walk to a park, this small playground next to a playfield may be for you. However, wooden climbing structures always present a risk of splinters, especially for children under two who need to hold on to the sides. The enclosed tube slide might be scary for a young toddler.

★★★½
ROBINSWOOD COMMUNITY PARK

24th Street and 148th Avenue SE, Bellevue

Access: Parking; stroller access

Features: Play equipment for tots (slides, swings, climbers, bouncers), woodchip play area surface, restrooms, some nursing privacy, shade

No changing table, no food or drink available

A delightful little duck pond is a short distance from the playground at Robinswood Community Park. The grassy area surrounding the pond is an ideal spot for a picnic lunch. Trees dapple the park and playground with shade. The playground provides enough excitement to keep your toddler busy and happy.

★★★½
WILBURTON HILL PARK

128th Avenue and 2nd Street NE, Bellevue

Access: Parking; stroller access

Features: Play equipment for tots (slides, swings, climbers, bouncer), woodchip play area surface, restrooms, food and drink in vending machine, nursing privacy, shade

no changing table

Large Wilburton Hill Park hosts trails, tennis courts, a botanical garden and a colorful playground. Look for the playground in the park's southeast corner. Five little playhouses sport smalltown names such as U.S. Post Office and General Store; climbers follow the same theme. A ladder and stairs help toddlers reach the top of the town hall. Youngsters can also climb in a wooden play ship, boat and railroad station. The restrooms and vending machines are a bit of a walk to the north.

Kirkland & Redmond

ANDERSON PARK (425)556-2300

7802 NE 168th Avenue, Redmond

Access: Parking; stroller access

Features: Play equipment for tots (slides, swings, climbers), pebble play area surface, restrooms, food and drink nearby, shade

No changing table, no nursing privacy

Located in the commercial area of Redmond, this park offers a fine resting point for picnicking and playing. A small playground adorns the southeastern tip of the park. Redmond Parks and Recreation uses quaint cottages in the park for classes.

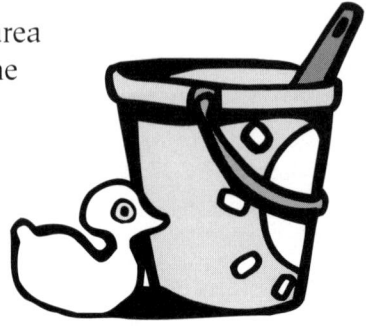

See the Anderson Park/Redmond Parks and Recreation description, page 108–109.

★★
CRESTWOOD PARK

6th Street and 18th Avenue, Kirkland

Access: Parking; stroller access

Features: Play equipment for tots (slides, swings, climbers, bouncers), woodchip play area surface, restrooms, limited nursing privacy, some shade

No changing table, no food or drink available

You will find the toddlers' play-lot at the northeast corner of Crestwood Park. The park also contains a number of hiking trails and a playfield. A high school uses the playfield, but the park appears big enough to accommodate everyone. There is ample parking.

★★
EVEREST PARK

8th Street and 5th Avenue S, Kirkland

Access: Parking; stroller access
Features: Play equipment for tots(swings, climbers, bouncers), woodchip play area surface, restrooms, nursing privacy, shade

No changing table, no food or drink available

At Everest Park the play-lot lies unshaded in the middle of a large playfield. A more serene place to visit is the wooded portion of the park by the north parking lot. Here trees lend shade to a small, quiet area bordering a narrow creek. A little bridge that crosses over the creek leads you to a path in the sunny center of the park.

★★★
FARRELL-MCWHIRTER PARK

19545 Redmond Road, Redmond

Access: Parking; stroller access
Features: Play equipment for tots (swings, climbers), sand play area surface, restrooms, nursing privacy, shade

No changing table, no food or drink available

This large park hosts a farm with pens for viewing a variety of farm animals. An expansive field is available for picnics or play. Take the trails that wind around the wooded portion of the park and stop at the play equipment down by the creek. Parking is a little distance from the farm, so you'll want to take your stroller.

★★
FORBES CREEK PARK

116th Place and 106th Lane NE, Kirkland

Access: Parking; stroller access
Features: Play equipment for tots (slides, swings, climbers), woodchip play area surface, shade

No restrooms. no changing table, no food or drink available, no nursing privacy

If you live in the Forbes Creek neighborhood you may want to visit this park. A quiet play-lot can be a perfect place to rest on a stroller walk. Nearby on 100th Street and 117th Place is Spinney Homestead Park, which you can also take in as part of a stroll around the neighborhood.

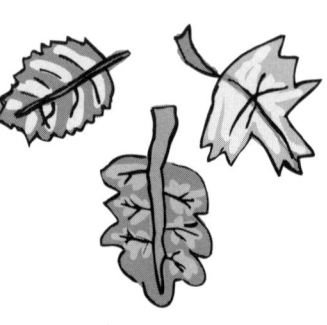

★★★
GRASS LAWN PARK

Old Redmond Way and 148th Avenue NE, Redmond

Access: Parking; stroller access
Features: Play equipment for tots (slides, climbers, swings), pebble play area surface, restrooms, nursing privacy, shade

No changing table, no food or drink available

Over twenty-eight acres of property make up this park with

the simple name. Of the park's two playgrounds, the one near the parking off Old Redmond Way has better equipment and better shade. In addition to playgrounds, the park includes sheltered picnic tables, open fields, trails and restrooms, making it perfect for families with children of all ages.

★★
HOUGHTON BEACH PARK

Lake Washington Boulevard and 60th Street NE, Kirkland

Access: Parking; stroller access

Features: Play equipment for tots (slides, climbers), woodchip play area surface, restrooms, food and drink, nursing privacy

No changing table, no shade

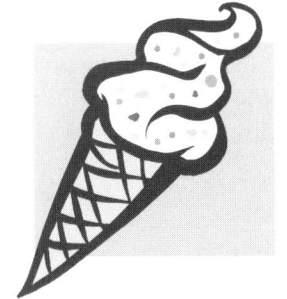

Sunshine, sand and lawn make up this waterfront park. There is little shade, so take sunscreen. The play lot is adequate for toddlers. Although the playground is located on a busy boulevard, a high fence keeps the little ones safe. Kidd Valley Hamburgers is across the street.

★★
IDYLWOOD PARK

38th Street and West Lake Sammamish Parkway NE, Redmond

Access: Parking; stroller access
Features: Restrooms, changing table, food and drink in vending machines, nursing privacy, shade

No play equipment for tots

This park located on Lake Sammamish is a fine spot for a

family outing. Not only is there a beach, but there are also woods and fields for those not interested in swimming. The parking lot is a bit far from the park, so take your stroller.

★★
JONATHAN HARTMAN PARK

17300 NE 104th Street, Redmond

Access: Parking; stroller access
Features: Play equipment for tots (slides, swings, climbers), woodchip play area surface, restrooms, changing table, shade

No food or drink available, no nursing privacy

Jonathan Hartman Park is located next to the Redmond swimming pool, and is across from Redmond High School. The park has ample shade near the playground. Ballfields that host little league games edge the western half of the parking lot.

★★½
JUANITA BAY PARK

Forbes Creek Drive and 98th Avenue NE, Kirkland

Access: Parking; stroller access
Features: Restrooms, nursing privacy, some shade

No play equipment for tots, no changing table, no food or drink available

Come sit under the beautiful willow trees and absorb nature with your little one. Take your stroller on the paved path through this reserve on

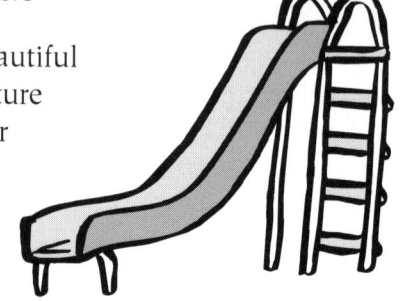

Juanita Bay. This tranquil locale should to be sought out if you love soft grass with a little shade. However, parking may be hard to find on a sunny day.

★★★★

MARYMOOR PARK

6046 NE West Lake Sammamish Parkway, Redmond

Access: Parking; stroller access
Features: Play equipment for tots (slides, swings, climbers, bouncers), woodchip play area surface, restrooms, nursing privacy, shade

No changing table, no food or drink available

A large windmill and totem pole welcome visitors to fascinating Marymoor Park. The beautiful grounds of Willowmoor Farm Historic District has a wealth of things for people of all ages to do. The Clise Mansion holds a museum of the history of the Eastside. The Marymoor Wetland Trail provides a pleasant walk through a wildlife preserve. 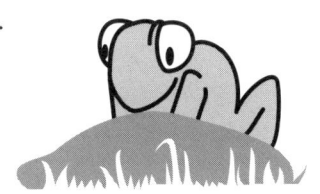 The Marymoor Velodrome is an exciting place to watch bicycles zooming by. If all that is not enough, a large playground is available for children of all ages to romp, run and climb until exhaustion. The Sammamish River Trail, which eventually becomes the Burke-Gilman Trail and runs into Seattle, begins at the park entrance.

Bringing Out Creepers, Crawlers & Toddlers • The Eastside

★★
MEADOW PARK

106th Street and 106th Avenue NE, Redmond

Access: Parking; stroller access
Features: Play equipment for tots (slides, climbers), dirt play area surface, shade

No restrooms. no changing table, no food or drink available, no nursing privacy

    This neighborhood park stands out for its well-shaded tot-lot. The playground is situated at the southwest corner of a rolling meadow. The paved pathway winds around the small park, so a summer evening stroll can easily end at the playground for some last-minute energy burn-off.

★★★★
NORTH KIRKLAND PARK

124th Street and 103rd Avenue NE, Kirkland

Access: Parking; stroller access
Features: Play equipment for tots (swings, climbers, bouncers), woodchip play area surface, restrooms, changing table, nursing privacy, shade

No food or drink available

    This bright, colorful playground is perfect for little acrobats. The climber's train theme gives the park its charm. Shaded grassy sections invite you to sit with your young baby. Across the street is the North Kirkland Community Center with activities for the little one. You will also find restrooms with changing tables at the center.
    See the North Kirkland Community Center description, page 116–117.

★★
PETER KIRK PARK

4th Street and Central Way NE, Kirkland

Access: Parking across the street, stroller access
Features: Play equipment for tots (slides, climbers), woodchip play area surface, restrooms, food and drink at Kirkland Park Place, some shade

No changing table, no nursing privacy

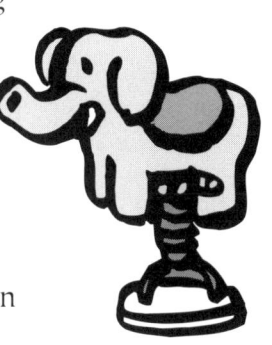

Visit Peter Kirk Park after shopping at Kirkland Park Place. The large downtown park has a playfield, benches and a playground. You can pick up some good food at Noah's Bagels or QFC Grocery and have a picnic while your little one crawls or toddles around on the grass. The Kirkland Library and Peter Kirk Pool are on the southwest corner of the park

★★½
SPIRITBROOK PARK

6500 NE 151st Avenue, Redmond

Access: Parking; stroller access
Features: Play equipment for tots (slides, climbers, swings, bouncers), pebble play area surface

No restrooms, no changing table, no food or drink available, no nursing privacy, no shade

This quaint playground won't intimidate young toddlers with its small climber and slide. However, the little pond is quite close to the playground and could become an attractive nuisance to inquisitive youngsters.

★★½

VAN AALST PARK

4th Street and 13th Avenue, Kirkland

Access: Parking; stroller access
Features: Play equipment for tots (slides, swings, climbers, bouncers), woodchip play area surface, little shade

No restrooms, no changing table, no food or drink available, no nursing privacy

You can't miss the fluorescent-colored climbing structure in this small triangular park. This quiet neighborhood park is fine for a walker or crawler. There is little shade for those younger babies to sit under.

★½

WAVERLY BEACH PARK

6th Street and Waverly Way W, Kirkland

Access: Parking; stroller access
Features: Restrooms, shade in morning hours

No play equipment for tots, no changing table, no food or drink available, no nursing privacy

This pretty beach park is best for immobile babies who cannot yet crawl. Instead of a sand bank, cement steps lead down into the water. I mention this beach because it is very attractive, but I would not want a crawler or walker getting too near the water. Large trees that border the park to the east lend morning shade.

★
WILLOWS CREEK PARK

8915 NE 142nd Avenue, Redmond

Access: Parking; stroller access
Features: Play equipment for tots (slides, climbers), woodchip play area surface, nursing privacy, shade

No restrooms, no changing table, no food or drink available

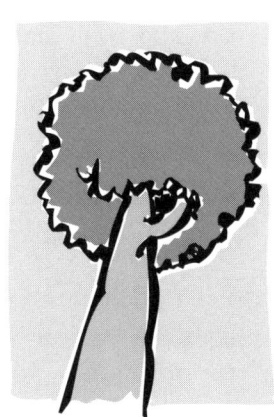

Willows Creek Park is at the end of 142nd Avenue off Redmond Way. The park's small playground lies next to a wooded area that is at the edge of a bluff. This is an adequate neighborhood playground, but not worth driving to from a distance.

Newcastle, Issaquah & Renton

★★★★
GENE COULON MEMORIAL BEACH PARK

1201 N Lake Washington Boulevard, Renton

Access: Parking; stroller access

Features: Play equipment for tots (slides, swings, climbers), sand play area surface, beach, restrooms, food and drink available, little nursing privacy, minimal shade

No changing table

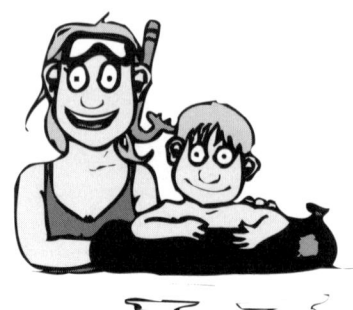

Spread along the southeast shore of Lake Washington, this park has beaches, playground, volleyball courts and more. There is plenty of fun to be had at this popular beach park. Pull into the South Beach parking lot if you want to be near the playground, then take your stroller for a walk to the pavilion, where you can pick up lunch at Ivar's or Kidd Valley.

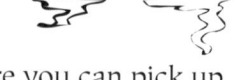

★★
KIWANIS PARK

815 NE Union Avenue, Renton

Access: Parking on 7th Avenue; stroller access on 7th Avenue

Features: Play equipment for tots (slides, swings, climbers), sand play area surface, nursing privacy, some shade

No changing table, no food or drink available

This playground sits across the street from an elementary

school. The City of Renton hosts a children's afterschool program in the park, so it can get busy in the late afternoon. Large evergreen trees provide shade for a grassy area on the southeast corner, but the playground is all sun, so take sunscreen.

★★★ ½
LAKE SAMMAMISH STATE PARK

Lake Sammamish Road and 17th Avenue NW, Issaquah

Access: Parking; stroller access

Features: Play equipment for tots (slides, climbers), sand play area surface, restrooms, food and drink, nursing privacy, shade

No changing table

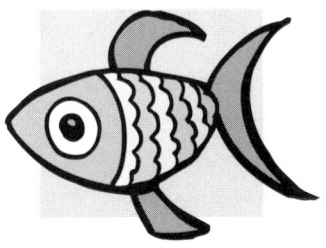

This large state preserve sits at the south end of Lake Sammamish. Besides an excellent public beach, this popular eastside destination has trails, picnic tables and volleyball nets. In summertime it becomes very busy. Although there are lots of shady spots, the playground and beach are quite sunny, so take plenty of sunscreen.

★★★
MEMORIAL PARK

140 E Sunset Way, Issaquah

Access: Parking; stroller access

Features: Play equipment for tots (slides, swings, climbers, bouncers), woodchip play area surface, restrooms in the library, nursing privacy, shade

No changing table, no food or drink available

Find this playground near the library and the Issaquah Train Depot Museum. The clean, colorful play equipment is a popular destination for toddlers. Shade, which dapples the playground, is deeper around the picnic benches and grass. Unfortunately, the only restrooms are in the library, which isn't open until 11 a.m.

★★
LAKE BOREN PARK

13000 SE 84th Way, Newcastle

Access: Parking; stroller access
Features: Play equipment for tots (slides, swings, climbers), woodchip play area surface, portable toilet, minimal nursing privacy

No changing table, no food or drink available, no shade

A paved walkway with ups and downs loops around Lake Boren Park, making it a great place for running with a stroller. Newer playground equipment is suitable for toddlers but the lack of shade makes sunscreen a must. A grassy field is perfect for romping and rolling.

★★★
LIBERTY PARK

Bronson Way N and Houser Way N, Renton

Access: Parking; stroller access
Features: Play equipment for tots (slides, swings, climbers, bouncers), woodchip play area surface, restrooms, nursing privacy, some shade

No changing table, no food or drink available

This large park is sandwiched between I–405 and Maple Valley Road, making it a bit noisy. The playground sports a large climbing structure as well as the other necessities for fun. A sunny field is available for running and romping or having a picnic. There are also plenty of picnic tables if that is more your preference. Located next to the Renton Public Library, this park makes a nice side trip after a library outing.

★★½
NEWCASTLE BEACH

4400 SE Lake Washington Boulevard, Newcastle

Access: Parking; stroller access
Features: Play equipment for tots (slides, swings, bouncers), woodchip play area surface, restrooms, nursing privacy, some shade

No changing table, no food or drink available

This twenty-nine acre park is located on Lake Washington. Shaded picnic benches next to the small sunny playground are close enough for you to sit while watching your toddler play. The swimming beach is perfect for little ones to stick their feet in the cold water without going too deep. If grassy fields are more your style, there is an open area for picnic blankets and relaxing.

★★★
THOMAS TEASDALE PARK
601 S 23rd, Renton

Access: Parking; stroller access
Features: Play equipment for tots (slides, climbers), sand play area surface, restrooms, food and drink available, nursing privacy, minimal shade

No changing table

The playground at Thomas Teasdale Park is better for older children since the climbers may be difficult for small children to use. However, there is plenty of grass to run around on and picnic tables in shelters if it rains.

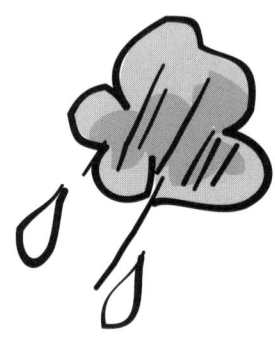

CHAPTER • THREE
Bringing OUT Baby Shopping & Dining

SHOPPING

GROCERY STORE PLAYROOMS

Some grocery stores in the Seattle offer free childcare within the store, in a playroom filled with toys and activities. Usually your child must be over two, but does not have to be potty-trained. If your child has a soiled diaper or starts to cry, the staff will page you over the intercom. Don't count on your baby co-operating every time; my toddler has wavered in his desire to use playrooms of this type. He refused for a long time, then for about a year he loved it, and suddenly his willingness to be left alone waned. If your child is eager, it is a wonderful way to handle grocery shopping. The following locations offer child care:

Fred Meyer–Bellevue (425)865–8560
2041 NE 148th Street, Bellevue

Fred Meyer–Burien (206)433–6411
14300 S First Avenue, Seattle

Fred Meyer–Benson Plaza (425)235–5350
17801 SE 108th Avenue, Renton

Fred Meyer–Covington (253) 639–7400
16735 SE 272nd Street, Kent

Fred Meyer–Federal Way (253) 952-0100
33702 SW 21st Avenue, Federal Way

Fred Meyer–Renton (425)204–5200
365 SW Renton Center Way, Renton

QFC–University Village (206)523–5160
2746 NE 45th Avenue, Seattle

Shopping Malls

Shopping malls are excellent spots to take baby when the weather is poor. From newborn to two years old, a young child loves the stimulation of people, colorful lights and the attractive window displays. Also, parents enjoy being among other adults while entertaining their young one at the same time. My son has always enjoyed going to the mall. Even at seventeen months he remained content just to ride in the stroller while I window-shopped.

Overall, Nordstrom has the best nursing areas of all the

stores. They usually provide a quiet room with comfortable couches and low lights. Changing tables are permanent fixtures, not the plastic pull-down type, which I never feel at ease using. The Bon Marché comes in a close second, but the rooms were not as private or cozy as at Nordstrom. J.C. Penney and Sears usually have plastic pull-down changing tables and there is no place to nurse comfortably. The best nursing area or changing table at the mall are noted first.

Under the food category I have concentrated on places that offered baby-friendly foods, although there may be other places in the mall to eat.

Most of the malls are equal in quality so I chose not to rate them. The comments can help you decide which one to visit.

ALDERWOOD MALL

184th Street and Alderwood Mall Boulevard SW, Lynnwood

Baby clothes: Gap Kids, Gymboree, Sears, Disney Store, Nordstrom, Bon Marché, J.C. Penney
Baby shoes: Stride Rite, J.C. Penney, Nordstrom
Toys: Kay Bee Toys, Disney Store, Imaginarium
Food: Food Court has pretzel, rice, chicken
Play area: None
Restrooms and changing tables: Nordstrom's ladies lounge is on the second floor opposite side from elevator. J.C. Penney's is on the first floor, by Customer Service; Bon Marché's is on the mall level by elevator and second floor by elevator; mall restrooms are in the food court
Nursing privacy: Nordstrom's ladies lounge has an area for nursing; Bon Marché's woman's restroom on second level

Alderwood Mall is a large shopping complex in Lynnwood. Target and Toys 'R Us, just outside the mall, are excellent for baby necessities. Target has a wide range of baby clothes and baby equipment. Toys 'R Us offers much more than just toys—you will find everything for babies from diapers to strollers there. To reach it, take the Alderwood Mall Exit off I-5.

BELLEVUE SQUARE

8th Street and Bellevue Way NE, Bellevue

Baby clothes: Gap Kids, Gymboree, Lil' People, Warner Bros. Studio Store, Nordstrom, Bon Marché, J.C. Penney, Disney Store
Baby shoes: Stride Rite, Kinney Shoes, Nordstrom, J.C. Penney
Toys: Warner Bros. Studio Store, FAO Schwartz, Great Train Store, Imaginarium, Sanrio Gift Gate, Disney Store
Food: Various restaurants, McDonalds
Play area: First level, East Common, in front of Eddie Bauer. Second level, East Common, near J.C. Penney
Restrooms and changing tables: Nordstrom's ladies lounge is on the second floor opposite side from elevator. J.C. Penney's is on the first floor, by Customer Service; Bon Marché's is on the mall level by elevator and second floor by elevator; Mall's "family restrooms" are on the first and second level by Nordstrom
Nursing privacy: Nordstrom's ladies lounge has an area for nursing. Bon Marché's woman's restroom mall level has chairs for nursing

Bellevue Square is the crème de la crème of malls in the Seattle area. It has the standard department stores as well as every chain store that offers childrens' items. During the Christmas season it is packed with hurrying shoppers. Even during other times of the year there are substantial numbers of shoppers spending time and money. The one down-side to this two-story shopping complex is the lack of convenient elevators. Only one elevator is located in the middle of the mall; another is to the west by the exit. Each department store has its own elevator as well, so use them when you find them. My favorite store in Bellevue Square is The Right Start. When I am too impatient to wait for a catalog order, I will go right to the source for interesting baby accessories.

Bellevue Square is located off I-405; take either the 8th Street or 4th Street exit.

CROSSROADS MALL

8th Street and 156th Avenue NE, Bellevue

Baby clothes: Kids Club, Old Navy, Lamonts
Baby shoes: Kids Club, Old Navy
Toys: Kids Club
Food: International flair, rice, roasted chicken
Play area: Coin-operated carousel, Playspace (may not be appropriate for children under two), Playspace (see page 119)
Restrooms and changing tables: Mall restrooms by Old Navy
Nursing privacy: None

The large food court is the central attraction of this mall. While you get a bite to eat, you little one will be entertained by watching the people eating at the multitude of tables that fill the center of the mall. You can find something for the most finicky eater from the wide selection of food. Old Navy, one of the few stores for babies at this mall, is noted for high quality, inexpensive baby clothes. Check out the socks—they do not slip off tiny feet and have little rubber traction grips on the soles. The mall's Playspace area is available to all children, but I find it inappropriate for children under three.

You will find Crossroads Mall on 156th Avenue and 8th Street; I take the 148th Street exit South off SR520, then turn east on NE 8th Street.

FACTORIA SQUARE

36th Street and 128th Avenue SE, Bellevue

Baby clothes: Mervyns, Lamonts,
Baby shoes: Target
Toys: Dream Tree Toys, Target
Food: Buffet, bakeries
Play area: Climbing structure that looks like a boat is outside of Dream Tree Toys
Restrooms and changing tables: Mall Women's restroom near Pearl Vision has a counter; Target
Nursing privacy: Women's restroom near Pearl Vision

This small mall is located in the southeast part of Bellevue. It has an arcade for older children, but it is not appropriate for toddlers and infants. Target is well stocked with all sorts of baby supplies. There is also a Pay-Less Drug Store and a Safeway Grocery store in this mall. To reach it, exit I-405 at Coal Creek Parkway South, turn left on SE Newport Way, and continue north on 128th Avenue SE.

GILMAN VILLAGE

Gilman Boulevard and Juniper Street NE, Issaquah

Baby clothes: Forget Me Not
Baby shoes: No
Food: Restaurants, candy, bakery
Toys: White Horse Toys, Anglomania/Cottontail Corner
Play area: See the First Steps description, pages 110–111.
Restrooms and changing tables: In mall restrooms
Nursing privacy: No

This quaint outdoor mall is comprised of historic homes and cottages renovated to hold stores and restaurants. Brick sidewalks and wood decking give the mall the feel of an old Northwest town. In addition to the shops listed above, there are interesting gift and jewelry stores that are fun to explore.

Check out the color displays at Sweet Additions, but prepared for a lot of "I want's" from your toddler.

LAKE FOREST PARK TOWNE CENTRE

17171 NE Bothell Way, Lake Forest Park

Baby clothes: Lamonts
Baby shoes: Lamonts
Food: Asian, Mexican, Burgers, Bakery
Toys: Tree Top Toys, Rite Aid, Third Place Books (book related)
Play area: In Third Place Books
Restrooms and changing tables: In Third Place Books restrooms
Nursing privacy: Yes, in children's section and couches in food court

On the second floor of the Lake Forest Park Towne Centre is Third Place Books where you will find a large food court in addition to a wonderful bookstore. The food court has enough variety to please any palate. Along with tables and chairs, couches are available for semi-private nursing. The bookstore offers new and used books and provides a children's section in the southeast corner. Soft beanbag chairs in the middle of this section offer another comfortable nursing area that will work well if you have an older child in tow. While you feed the baby, your other child can read books or play with blocks provided in baskets on the floor near you.

NORTHGATE MALL

Northgate Way and 5th Avenue NE, North Seattle

Baby clothes: Gap Kids, Gymboree, Nordstrom, Bon Marché, J.C. Penney, Lamonts, Disney Store
Baby shoes: Nordstrom, J.C. Penney, The Athlete's Foot, Foot Action USA
Food: Red Robin, hamburgers, Asian food
Toys: Toys R' Us, Disney Store, Learning Smith

Play area: None
Restrooms and changing tables: Nordstrom second floor by Town Square; J.C. Penney first floor by lingerie; Bon Marché ground floor level by the lingerie department and second floor by linen department
Nursing privacy: Nordstrom ladies lounge has an area for nursing; Bon Marché's women's lounge second floor; J.C.

Northgate Mall is the very first shopping mall, after which others in the U.S. were patterned. It is smaller than Bellevue Square and Southcenter, but still has most of what one expects to find in this type of shopping complex. An extensive renovation updated this mall, adding a food court at the south end. The Red Robin restaurant is loud and full of families at anytime so there are plenty of distractions for your impatient toddler. On the northern end of this mall is Northgate Theater, which offers a crying room for parents attending movies. See page 61 for a description. Northgate is off I-5, on the east side of the freeway; an exit for the mall is marked.

REDMOND TOWNE CENTER

Leary Way and 76th Avenue, Redmond

Baby clothes: Baby Gap, Boston Baby Store, Brat Pack
Baby shoes: Baby Gap, Brat Pack
Food: Hamburgers, coffee, cookies, Mexican
Toys: K.B. Toys, Dream Tree
Play area: In front of K.B. Toys
Restrooms and changing tables: In mall restrooms on north side, ground level
Nursing privacy: No

This outdoor mall offers two levels of shops and restaurants. Covering over the aisles of shops provides rain protection. A street runs through the center of the mall, so watch your toddlers. Near the Starbucks is an active water fountain in which your kids can play, so dress them in shorts and sandals. The Dream Tree offers high quality toys such as Thomas the Tank Engine®, Brio®, and Playmobile®. There is plenty of covered parking.

Kid's Cut 'N Play, located on the top floor of the central parking lot, a haircut salon geared to youngsters, offers drop-in care for children over two. Call (425)869-2527 for information.

SOUTHCENTER MALL

Southcenter Parkway and Tukwila Parkway, Tukwila

Baby clothes: Gap Kids, Gymboree, Nordstrom, Bon Marché, J.C. Penney, Sears, Disney Store, Limited for Kids
Baby shoes: Stride Rite, Nordstrom, J.C. Penney
Food: Food court has bread, rice, chicken
Toys: Kay Bee Toys, Disney Store, Imaginarium, Character Corner
Play area: Arcade with tot rides
Restrooms and changing tables: Nordstrom ladies' lounge and men's room third floor and second floor; J.C. Penney second floor; Bon Marché second floor; Sears second floor; Mall restrooms in the food court
Nursing privacy: Nordstrom's ladies' lounge third floor has a pleasant nursing area; Bon Marché's ladies' lounge also has a nice area for nursing

Southcenter Mall is a large shopping mall in an even larger shopping district just south of Seattle. This area in Tukwila is known for its large variety of furniture stores. Most of the chain retail stores have a spot here at Southcenter.

You will easily find the mall in the southeast quadrant of the I–405/I–5 interchange. Both freeways have a Southcenter Mall exit.

UNIVERSITY VILLAGE

45th Street and 25th Avenue NE, Laurelhurst

Baby clothes: Baby Gap, Kids Club
Baby shoes: Baby Gap, Shoe Zoo
Food: QFC Grocery, bagels, wraps, bakery
Toys: Kids Club, Bartell Drugs, Channel 9 Store, Go To Your Room
Play area: Small gated area with toddler toys and climbers; Closed 9–10 a.m. and 3–4 p.m.
Restrooms and changing tables: Barnes and Noble
Nursing privacy: None

University Village is an excellent place to come for most of your shopping needs. It is an outside mall, so come prepared in inclement weather. However, there is enough cover over the promenade that you will not need an umbrella. A small tot play area in the middle of the mall is a fine place for your toddler to let off steam before going into another store. Life-sized sculptures of a cow and calf, which always attract youngsters, pay homage to the time when this property was part of a Carnation milk bottling plant. In front of the Channel 9 Store is a stone water sculpture that children can play in, although it may be a bit much for toddlers.

QFC has a child-care room available for children over two. Barnes and Noble bookstore alone is worth the trip to University Village. This huge store has a wonderful selection of children's books and has a storyteller Fridays at 11:00 a.m.

Go To Your Room, on the far north side of the shopping center, specializes in children's furniture and storage, and carries a small selection of toys.

Just north of the University Village on Blakely Street, which turns into Union Bay Place, you'll find the Right Start, Pinocchio Toys, and All for Kids.

WALLINGFORD CENTER/NORTH 45th STREET

45th Street and Wallingford Avenue N, Wallingford

Baby clothes: Boston Street Baby Store, Kids on 45th (new and used clothes)
Baby shoes: Kids on 45th
Food: QFC, bagels
Toys: Imagination Toys
Play area: First floor Wallingford Center, Kids on 45th
Restrooms and changing tables: No
Nursing privacy: None

Boston Street Baby Store has a wide selection of colorful cotton baby clothes and baby accessories. Although Imagination Toys is a small store, it is stocked to the brim with unique and perennial favorites. This store has higher quality toys that you may not find at Toys R' Us. Across the street at Kids on 45th you'll find used baby clothes, shoes and toys as well as new accessories. If groceries are needed, just walk over to the brand new QFC grocery store that has a natural food section on the second floor.

Restaurants

Taking babies (and toddlers especially) to a restaurant can be a trying experience. However, when both parents have worked all day inside or outside the home, cooking can be a low priority. Dining out has become a necessity of a hectic life. The restaurants I investigated welcome babies and toddlers. Most furnish crayons or toys to entertain a child, and offer children's menus with smaller portions at cheaper prices.

I have not rated the restaurants since I do not have a discriminating palate. I do provide brief descriptions of the types of food and the price ranges of the adult and children's menus. I placed restaurants with Multiple Locations in the beginning, then divide the rest by neighborhood in Seattle, and city on the Eastside.

Even at the most accommodating restaurants, it may seem to be impossible to dine out with your toddler, but don't be discouraged. Keep on eating out; with time your child should be able to dine at a restaurant without embarrassing his parents too much. When my son was two, we thought we would have to give up restaurants forever. Finally, at age three we get complimented on his restaurant behavior.

There are a few things you can do to make dining a little easier. First, bring a toddler who is hungry, but not too hungry. A child who is not hungry will quickly become restless, but one who is too hungry won't be able to wait until the food comes. Be sure to bring Cheerios to occupy little hands and mouth before the food comes. Second, let your child pick out some small toys from home to play with on the table while you wait for your food. Finally, be prepared to walk a restless child around the restaurant or outside before the food comes or while waiting for the check. If you expect this, you won't be annoyed when your meal has to be rushed to accommodate your child.

Multiple Locations

CUCINA! CUCINA! ITALIAN CAFÉ

Most toddlers love spaghetti, and this restaurant chain has plenty of it. Every parent I've spoken with has suggested Cucina! Cucina! for dining with small children. The menu, from spaghetti in red sauce to the more interesting pasta combinations, appeals to everyone. Children enjoy playing with the complimentary crayons and they also receive a glob of pasta dough to entertain them while the food is prepared.

901 N Fairview Avenue, Lake Union	(206)44-PASTA
800 NE Bellevue Way, #18, Bellevue	(425)637–1177
16499 NE 74th Street #E255, Redmond	(425)558–2200
1510 NW 11th Avenue, Issaquah	(425)391–3800
2031 S 316th Street, Federal Way	(253) 941–4800
2220 Carillon Point, Kirkland	(425)288–4000

RED ROBIN RESTAURANTS

The whole family will enjoy eating at Red Robin. This family-oriented restaurant is so full of kids that they can watch each other for entertainment. The menu includes sandwiches, salads, burgers and more. During lunch and dinner hours Red Robin can get crowded, which is entertaining if you are already seated, but can be a problem if you have to wait with your toddler.

3272 E Furman Avenue, Lake Union	(206)323-0918
1100 Fourth Avenue, Downtown	(206)447-1909
1101 Alaskan Way, Seattle	(206)447-1909
138 Northgate Plaza, Northgate	(206)365-0933
11021 NE 8th Street, Bellevue	(425)453-9522
1085 Lake Drive, Issaquah	(425)313-0950
2390 148th Street, Redmond	(425)641-3810
2233 S 320th Street, Federal Way	(253) 946-8646

WORLD WRAPPS

Snuggled into shopping districts, this chain has a variety of burrito-style entries, ranging from Thai wraps with peanut sauce to Mexican wraps with salsa. The children's menu offers smaller versions for smaller appetites. Crayons or toys aren't provided, but the colorful décor and bustling atmosphere will entertain youngsters. Waiting in line to order your food can pose a problem for impatient toddlers, so it is wise to have another adult sit with your child at a table while you wait for your order, especially during peak eating hours. Many of the locations are in shopping districts and provide a welcome respite from lugging a hungry toddler around while shopping.

1109 Madison Street, First Hill	(206)467-9744
528 N Queen Anne Avenue, Queen Anne	(206)286-9727
406 East Broadway, Capitol Hill	(206)328-9727
222 N Yale Avenue, Downtown	(206)233-0222
7900 E Green Lake Drive North, Suite 107, Green Lake	
	(206)524-9727

124 S Lake Street, Kirkland (425)827-9727
2750 NE University Village, Laurelhurst (206)522-7873

QUEEN ANNE

5 SPOT CAFÉ (206)285-7768
1502 N Queen Anne Avenue, Queen Anne

Access: Street parking; stroller access
Hours: Monday–Sunday 8:30 a.m.–12 a.m.
Menu: Pasta, sandwiches $8–$14, children's menu $3.25–$4.75
Features: Crayons and toys, changing table

This café, in the heart of Queen Anne on Queen Anne Avenue, has a diner atmosphere. The menu offers home-cooking entrees such as brisket and Jewish fare including borscht and knishes.

McGRAW STREET BAKERY CAFÉ (206)284-6327
615 W McGraw Street, Queen Anne

Access: Street parking; stroller access
Hours: Monday–Saturday 7 a.m.–5 p.m., Sunday 8 a.m.–4:30 p.m.
Menu: Pizza, soups, sandwiches $2–$4
Features: Children's books

No changing table

The small dining area for this Queen Anne bakery resembles a peaceful living room. Your toddler can sit at a small child's table nestled in the corner by the window and nibble on sprinkled cookies, while you enjoy a cup of coffee. Dim lighting and upholstered chairs in the rear provide a quiet place to nurse your baby.

Downtown

IRON HORSE RESTAURANT (206)223-9506

311 S 3rd Avenue, Downtown

Access: Parking in pay lot on 2nd Avenue; stroller access
Hours: Sunday–Friday 11 a.m.–7 p.m., Saturday 11 a.m.–8 p.m.
Menu: American, $5–$9, children's menu $4–$5.50
Features: Crayons and toys

No changing table

Bring young train enthusiasts to see their food delivered by model trains running on tracks that flank both sides of the restaurant. A train whistle blows every time a train leaves the kitchen and toddlers pop up from their seats and wait to see the train run. If there are many diners, trains are going back and forth throughout your meal. Model trains exhibited on the walls, along with photos and posters of trains, complete the atmosphere.

IVAR'S ACRES OF CLAMS (206)624-6852

1001 Alaskan Way, Pier 54, Downtown

Access: Parking; stroller access
Hours: Daily 11 a.m.–11 p.m.
Menu: Seafood $13–$30, children's menu $3–$5,
Features: Crayons and toys

No changing table,

Ivar's is a Seattle tradition for clam chowder and seafood. Request a table by the window so your child can look out on the fireboat docked next door. Both long-time residents and tourists frequent this restaurant on the waterfront near the Pike Place Market. Be sure to visit the Seattle Aquarium or the Bay Carousel while you're in the area.

Ravenna & Laurelhurst

BAGEL OASIS (206)526-0525

2112 NE 65th Street, Ravenna

Access: Parking; stroller access
Hours: Monday–Friday 6 a.m.–5 p.m., Saturday and Sunday 7 a.m.–4 p.m.
Menu: Sandwiches, omelets $1–$5.95
Features: Changing table

No crayons or toys

Bagels are perfect for toddlers. They come in many flavors that can satisfy even the pickiest eater. The casual atmosphere at the Bagel Oasis provides an easy lunch or breakfast for you and your little one, and the menu is broad enough to satisfy your appetite as well as your child's.

THE ROASTED PEPPER (206)525–6500

3701 NE 45th Street

Access: Parking; stroller access
Hours: Monday–Saturday 8 a.m.–9 p.m., Sunday 8 a.m.–8 p.m.
Menu: American $5–$10, children's menu $3.50–$3.95
Features: Crayons

No changing table,

The Roasted Pepper's big dining room is perfect for large families sharing single pizzas, or looking for reasonably priced dinners of salads, wraps, sandwiches and entrees. Since breakfast, lunch and dinner are served daily, this restaurant is a convenient choice.

NORTHGATE, WALLINGFORD & GREEN LAKE

THE BELLS (206)524-3100

8502 NE 5th Avenue, Northgate

Access: Parking; stroller access
Hours: Monday–Friday 11 a.m.–8 p.m., Saturday 8 a.m.–8 p.m., Sunday 8 a.m.–7 p.m.
Menu: American $7.95–$10.95, children's menu $2.50–$2.95,
Features: Crayons and toys

No changing table,

This old-time Seattle restaurant is famous for its delicious pies. It is family oriented, with standard American fare. Filled with booths, it has the atmosphere of a diner offering old fashioned home cooking.

EGG CETERA'S BLUE STAR CAFÉ (206)548-0345

4512 N Stone Way, Wallingford

Access: Parking minimal; stroller access
Hours: Monday–Thursday 7 a.m.–3 p.m. and 5–10 p.m., Friday 7 a.m.–3 p.m. and 5 p.m.–11 p.m., Saturday 8 a.m.–3 p.m. and 5 p.m.–11 p.m., Sunday 8 a.m.–3 p.m. and 5 p.m.–10 p.m.
Menu: American, breakfasts $5.50–7.95, children's menu $2.25–$2.95 ,
Features: Crayons

No changing table,

This restaurant is best for families during breakfast and lunch hours. In the evenings the pub is open, which creates a more adult atmosphere. Breakfasts are reasonably priced and are very popular on weekends. The only drawback is that parking is difficult.

JULIA'S IN WALLINGFORD (206)633-1175

4401 N 45th Street, Wallingford

Access: Parking; stroller access
Hours: Monday–Thursday 7 a.m.–9p.m., Friday and Saturday 7 a.m.–10 p.m., Sunday 7:30 a.m.–9 p.m.
Menu: American $7–$13, children's menu
Features: Crayons and toys

No changing table,

Julia's supplies quick service, which is essential when dining with young children. Early evenings are best for fast seating, but expect to wait for Saturday and Sunday brunch. The children's menu has a lot of fried food, but the adult menu offers salads, sandwiches and vegetarian dinner entrees.

ZOKA COFFEE ROASTER AND TEA COMPANY
(206)545-4277

2200 N 56th Street, Green Lake

Access: Parking; stroller access
Hours: Open Monday–Saturday 6 a.m.- 12 a.m., Sunday 6 a.m.–10 p.m.
Menu: Baked goods, sandwiches $1.25–4.75
Features: Toys

No changing table

Check the rear of this Green Lake coffeehouse for a box full of toys. Good-mannered toddlers can eat cookies or muffins while you sip on coffee or tea. Comfortable sofas are available for relaxing with a calm infant. Saturday and Sunday mornings are very popular, so expect a short wait.

FREMONT, PHINNEY RIDGE & BALLARD

BARLEE'S FAMILY PIZZA AND PASTA   (206)633-4545

3410 NW Fremont Avenue, Fremont

Access: Street parking; stroller access
Hours: Monday–Friday 11:30 a.m.–9 p.m., Saturday and Sunday 8:30 a.m.–11 p.m.
Menu: Pizza, pasta, sandwiches $5.95–$9.95, children's menu $3.25
Features: Crayons

No changing table

Located in the heart of the Fremont district, Barlee's offers a variety of pasta, salads and entrees. If you find parking, be sure to take your stroller so you can visit the interesting shops on Fremont Avenue.

PESCATORE FISH CAFÉ   (206)784-1733

5300 NW 34th Avenue, Ballard

Access: Parking; stroller access
Hours: Monday–Thursday 11:30 a.m.–3 p.m. and 4:30–9:30 p.m., Friday 11:30 a.m.–3 p.m. and 4:30–10:30 p.m., Saturday 10:30 a.m.–3:00 p.m. and 4:30–10:30 p.m., Sunday 11:30 a.m.–3 p.m. and 4:30–9:30 p.m.
Menu: Seafood $8.95–$15.95, children's menu $2.95
Features: Crayons and toys, changing table

This swank, waterfront restaurant is a perfect place to take out-of-town visitors and your toddler to dinner. The menu offers typical Northwest fare and the children's menu provides more than just hot dogs and hamburgers. A toy basket filled with books, puzzles and toys can be brought back to your table to entertain your youngster before the food is served.

SANTA FE CAFÉ   (206)783-9755

5910 N. Phinney Avenue, Phinney Ridge

Access: Minimal parking in the back; stroller access
Hours: Monday–Friday 5–11 p.m., Saturday and Sunday 11–4 p.m. and 4–11 p.m.
Menu: New Mexican $8.95–$10.95, children's menu, $1.50–$5.50
Features: Crayons and toys

No changing table

The Santa Fe Café has an interesting variety of southern dishes. Fortunately, children are welcome and are always present. If your toddler gets too antsy sitting through an entire meal, one of your dinner party members can take the restless little one across the street to Woodland Park playground.

WEST SEATTLE

LUNA PARK CAFÉ   (206)935-7250

2910 SW Avalon Way, West Seattle

Access: Parking; stroller access
Hours: Daily 7 a.m.–11 p.m.
Menu: American $4.95–$6.95, children's menu $2.50–$2.95
Features: Crayons and toys

No changing table,

The walls of this funky café are decorated with colorful posters and pictures reminiscent of a 1950's restaurant where you can get a good burger and shake. Coin-operated machines will entertain youngsters. The

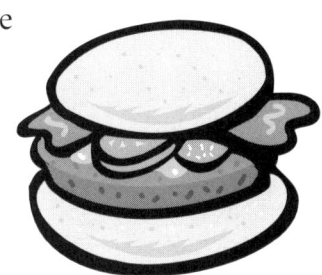

children's menu is varied enough to give a picky eater something that satisfies.

PEGASUS PIZZA AND PASTA (206)932-4849
2758 SW Alki Avenue, West Seattle

Access: Street parking; stroller access
Hours: Monday–Friday 11:30 a.m.–11 p.m., Saturday and Sunday 12–11 p.m.
Menu: Entreés, pasta $5.25–$8.25, children's menu $2.25–$3.00
Features: Crayons

No changing table

Located on Puget Sound, this popular West Seattle family pizzeria offers a wide variety of pizzas from Greek style with feta, spinach and olives to Italian sausage with mushrooms.

THE POINT GRILL (206)933-0118
2770 SW Alki Avenue, West Seattle

Access: Street parking; stroller access
Hours: Monday–Thursday 11 a.m.–9 p.m., Friday 11 a.m.–10 p.m., Saturday 12–10 p.m. and Sunday 12–9 p.m.
Menu: Traditional American $6.75–$14.75, children's menu, $3.25–$3.95
Features: Crayons

No changing table,

Look out over Puget Sound while enjoying lunch or dinner at the Point Grill. More children dine in this restaurant on the weekends, but younger preschoolers can be found here during weekdays. An interesting menu for moms and dads makes dining here an enjoyable experience.

BELLEVUE

BILLY McHALE'S RESTAURANT   (425)746-1138
4065 SE 128th Avenue, Bellevue

Access: Parking; stroller access
Hours: Monday–Thursday and Sunday 11 a.m.–9 p.m., Friday and Saturday 11 a.m.–10 p.m.
Menu: American, ribs Price Range: $5.95–$13.95 children's menu, $3.50–$4.50, crayons and toys, changing table

This family-oriented restaurant has a kid's corner play-space in the waiting area with a small television, crayons and toys to entertain your youngster while you wait for a table. You can take an impatient toddler there while the rest of the family eats dinner. I visited the location in Factoria, but there are also locations in Renton, Federal Way, Redmond, Alderwood and Lakewood.

COYOTE CREEK PIZZA COMPANY   (425)746-7460
15600 NE 8th Street, Bellevue

Access: Parking; stroller access
Hours: Monday–Thursday 11 a.m.–9 p.m., Friday 11 a.m.–11 p.m., Saturday 12–11 p.m., Sunday 12–9 p.m.
Menu: Pizza $3.95–$19.95

No crayons or toys, no changing table,

Although there are no crayons or children's menus, this pizza restaurant is popular with families. The exciting noises and southwestern flair help keep little eyes busy while you wait for your meal. The pizzas range from cheese to more exotic Thai or cracked crab. You may want to grab a take-out menu for those times you just can't get everyone together to go out. Look for this restaurant in Crossroads Mall near the movie theater.

Redmond & Issaquah

DESERT FIRE   (425)895-1500

7211 NE 166th Avenue, Redmond

Access: Parking; stroller access
Hours: Monday–Thursday and Sunday 11a.m.–10 p.m., Friday and Saturday 11 a.m.–11 p.m.
Menu: Southwestern $7–$13, children's menu $3.50
Features: Crayons and stickers, changing table

Park your family around the fire pit during a cold and rainy evening or dine on the patio in the summer. Whatever the weather you can enjoy Southwestern fare at this Redmond Town Center restaurant. The kids' menu, which includes burgers and spaghetti as well as southwestern standards, provides enough variety for the most finicky palates.

THE FISHIN' PLACE   (425)556-5900

17181 Redmond Way, Redmond

Access: Parking; stroller access
Hours: Daily 11 a.m.–8 p.m.
Menu: Fish, sushi $3.59–$9.59

No crayons or toys, no changing table,

If your trying to get your toddler to eat fish you'll want to take him to this take-out restaurant. The fun begins upon entering, as you walk over a short bridge that crosses running water. Once inside, your toddler will enjoy the fun and fishy décor as you pick out ready-made meals to take home and pop in your oven.

FRANKIE'S PIZZA (425)883-8407

16630 Redmond Way, Redmond

Access: Parking; stroller access
Hours: Monday–Thursday 11 a.m.–9:30 p.m., Friday 11 a.m.–11 p.m., Saturday 11 a.m.–10 p.m., Sunday 4–9 p.m.
Menu: Pizza, calzone, pasta $4.95–$12.95, children's menu $2.75–$4.25
Features: Crayons, changing table

Black and white checked tiles create a charming pizzeria atmosphere in this Redmond restaurant. Your toddler will enjoy the bright lights and lively décor while munching on fresh pizza. Or your family can savor the pasta, calzones or sandwiches.

JAY BERRY'S (425)392-0808

385 NW Gilman Boulevard, Issaquah

Access: Parking; no stroller access
Hours: Monday–Thursday 11 a.m.–10 p.m., Friday 11 a.m.–11 p.m., Saturday 12–11 p.m., Sunday 4–10 p.m.
Menu: Pizza, pasta, sandwiches $1.75–$11.95, children's menu, $1–$4.95
Features: Crayons and toys

No changing table

What's great about Jay Berry's is that it has tables against large windows that look out onto a creek. Children love to watch fish bobbing through the rapids as they wait for their meal. The kid's menu includes pastas, meatballs and even fish and chips, or you can order a pizza for the whole family.

JITTERS (425)747-8030

15010 NE 20th Avenue, Redmond

Access: Parking; stroller access
Hours: Monday–Friday 6:30 a.m.–730 p.m., Saturday 7 a.m.–7:30 p.m., Sunday 8:30 a.m.–6 p.m.
Menu: Coffee, pastries $0.75–$2.25
Features: Kids' climbing structure

No changing table

Sip lattés and munch one of a variety of pastries while your child enjoys a plastic climbing structure or flips through picture books. You will be able to keep an eye on toddlers as they play in a separate room with a large window. There are also highchairs suitable for infants so you don't have to keep your baby in the car seat while you eat.

KIRKLAND

BAGEL OASIS (425)823-5404

9805 NE 116th Street, Kirkland

Access: Minimal parking in the back; stroller access
Hours: Monday–Friday 6 a.m.–4 p.m., Saturday and Sunday 7 a.m.–4 p.m.
Menu: Breakfasts, sandwiches $1.75–$5.95
Features: Crayons and toys

No changing table

This restaurant offers reasonably priced food in a quaint café atmosphere. As you enter, a cozy nook to the left holds a low coffee table and two upholstered chairs that make a discrete place to nurse. This nook is also perfect for toddlers, since it is off from the main dining area and there is a basket filled with toys and books for youngsters.

BROWN BAG CAFÉ (425)822-9462

12217 NE 116th Street, Kirkland

Access: Parking; stroller access
Hours: Daily 6 a.m.–3 p.m.
Menu: Breakfasts, sandwiches $5.50–$7.75, children's menu $3.99, crayons and toys

No changing table

This popular family-style restaurant is especially busy on weekends. A Kirkland favorite for breakfast and lunch, the Brown Bag Café offers a large variety of breakfast items, sandwiches and salads. The children's menu is limited, but all lunch and breakfast items are $3.99.

CIRCO CIRCO (425)821-9405

12709 NE 124th Street, Kirkland

Access: Parking; stroller access
Hours: Monday–Thursday 11 a.m.–9 p.m., Friday and Saturday 11 a.m.- 10 p.m.
Menu: Mexican $4.95–$10.95, children's menu $1.75–$2.50 , crayons and toys

No changing table

Located in the Totem Place strip mall, which is across the street from Kirland Toyota, this restaurant is easy to miss. Look for it next to the Lucky 7 Saloon. Inside, the colorful circus décor will widen the eyes of your baby. Crayons, stickers and books will keep little fingers busy while you are waiting for food. Go for a birthday and get a special birthday treat for desert.

Quick Reference Guide

Top Ten Indoor Locations

First Steps (page 111) (425)392-2095
317 NW Gilman Boulevard, #9, Issaquah

Gymboree (page 24)
5001 NE 50th Street, Laurelhurst (206)522-2045
9250 NW 14thAvenue, Crown Hill (206)523-8011

Issaquah Community Center (page 112–113) (425)837-3300
301 S Rainier Boulevard, Issaquah

The Little Gym (page 57–58, 114–115)
7777 15th Avenue NE, Lake City (206)524-2623
1800 130th Avenue NE, Bellevue (425)885-3866

Loyal Heights Community Center
(page 58–59) (206)684-4052
2101 NW 77th Street, Loyal Heights

Quick Reference Guide

North Kirkland Community Center
(page 116–117) (425)828-1105
12421 NE 103rd Avenue, Kirkland

Pacific Science Center (page 36) (206)443-2880
200 N Second Avenue, Seattle Center

Playspace at Crossroads Mall
(page 119) (425)644-4500
Bellevue 4555 Delridge Way SW, West Seattle

Renton Community Center (page119–120) (425)235-2560
1715 Maple Valley Highway, Renton

Southwest Family Center (page94–95) (206)937-7680
4555 Delridge Way SW, West Seattle

Top Ten Outdoor Locations

Bitter Lake Park (page 73)
130th Street and Linden Avenue, Bitter Lake

Gene Coulon Memorial Beach Park (page 142)
1201 N Lake Washington Boulevard, Renton

Green Lake Park (page 70–71)
7201 E Green Lake Drive, Green Lake

Lake Hills Park (page 128)
14th Street and 164th Avenue, Bellevue

Lincoln Park (page 106)
8400 SW Fauntleroy Way, West Seattle

Marymoor Park (page 137)
6046 West Lake Sammamish Parkway NE, Redmond

North Kirkland Park (page 138)
124th Street and 103rd Avenue NE, Kirkland

Robinswood Community Park (page 131)
24th Street and 148th Avenue SE, Bellevue

Volunteer Park (page 40)
Prospect Street and 14th Avenue East, Capitol Hill

Woodland Park Zoo (page 86–87)
601 North 59th Street, Green Lake

Program For Early Parent Support (Peps)
Parent/Child Activity Time

Ballard Family Center (page 49)   (206)706-9645
5449 NW Ballard Avenue, Ballard

Bitter Lake Family Center (page 50–51)   (206)368-0172
13035 N Linden Avenue, Bitter Lake

Family Works (page 54–55)   (206)694-6727
1501 N 45th Avenue, Wallingford

Garfield Family Center (page 39)   (206)461-4486
Garfield Community Center, 2323 East Cherry Street, Central

Meadowbrook Family Center (page 60)   (206)366-9256
10517 35th Avenue NE, Lake City

North Seattle Family Support Center (page 62)
13540 NE Lake City Way, Suite 5, Lake City   (206)364-7930

Rainier Family Support Center (page 94)   (206)723-8590
Rainier Community Center, 4600 38th Avenue S, South Seattle

Southwest Family Center (page 94–95)   (206)937-7680
4555 Delridge Way SW, West Seattle

Movement Classes

Anderson Park (page 108–109)   (425)556-2300
7802 NE 168th Avenue, Redmond
Teenie Weenie Wigglers (2–3 years)

Gymboree (page 24–25)
5001 NE 50th Street, Laurelhurst   (206)522-2045
9250 14th Avenue NW, Crown Hill   (206)523-8011
2331 NE 140th Avenue, Bellevue   (425)392-8438
3302 E Lake Sammamish Parkway, Issaquah   (425)392-8438
33633 S 9th Avenue, Federal Way   (253) 661-7205

Gymbabies (1–5 months), Gymmovers (6–12 months), Bugs (4–10 months), Gymrunner (14–30 months), Gymexplorers (24–38 months)

Issaquah Community Center (page 112–113) (425)837-3300
301 S Rainier Boulevard, Issaquah
Little Gym (19–27 months), Little Gym (27–36 months)

The Little Gym (page 57–58, 92–93, 114–115)
7777 15th Avenue NE, Lake City   (206)524-2623
1800 130th Avenue NE, Bellevue   (425)885-3866

Birds (10–19 months), Beasts (19–30 months)

Magnolia Community Center (page 35–36) (206)362-7447
2550 W 34th Avenue, Magnolia

Tot Bop (1½ –3½ years), Baby Bop (under 18 months)

North Kirkland Community Center (page 116–117)
12421 NE 103rd Avenue, Kirkland (425)828-1105

Baby Bop (under 18 months), Parent/Toddler Movement (12–18 months), Parent/Child Movement (18–30 months), Preschool Movement (2½–3 years)

Northwest Center (page 118) (425)462-6046
9825 NE 24th Street

Romp and Roll (18–30 months)

Renton Community Center (page 119–120) (425)235-2560
1715 Maple Valley Highway, Renton

Toddlersize (2–3 years)

Seattle Gymnastics Academy (page 64–65) (206)386-4235
12535 NE 26th Avenue, Lake City

Parent/Tot Class (18–36 months)

University Family YMCA (page 68) (206)524-8613
5003 12th Avenue NE, University District

Parent/Tot Class (18–36 months)

Music Classes

Anderson Park (page 108–109) (425)556-2300
7802 NE 168th Avenue, Redmond

Kindermusik Beginnings (1½–3 years), Kindermusik Villages (newborn –18 months)

Ballard Family Center (page 49)　　　(206)706-9645
5449 NW Ballard Avenue, Ballard
Kindermusik (0–18 months)

Kindermusik Beginnings (page 25)　　1-800-628-5687 for a
(1½ and up)　　　　　　　　　　　　　location near you

Magnolia Community Center (page 35–36)　(206)386-4235
2550 34th Avenue West, Magnolia
Tot Bop (1½–3½ years), Baby Bop (under 18 months)

North Kirkland Community Center (page 116–117)
12421 NE 103rd Avenue, Kirkland　　　(425)828-1105
Music Makers and Shakers (2 years)

Northwest Center (page 118)　　　　(425)462-6046
9825 NE 24th Street, Bellevue
Kindermusik Beginnings (1½–2½ years), Musical Magic (1½–2½ years), Kindermusik Villages (newborn–18 months)

Ravenna-Eckstein Community Center (page 62–63)
6535 Ravenna Avenue NE, Ravenna　　(206)684-7534
Music Exploration (2–3 years)

Renton Community Center (page 119–120)　(425)235-2560
1715 Maple Valley Highway, Renton
Kindermusik Villages (newborn–18 months)

Tune Tales (page 67–68)　　　　　　(425)775-0608
John's Music, 4501 N Interlake, Wallingford

Quick Reference Guide

Arts and Crafts

Anderson Park (page 108–109)   (425)556-2300
7802 NE 168th Avenue, Redmond
Rainbow Makers (1½–3 years)

First Steps (page 110–111)   (425)392-2095, page
317 NW Gilman Boulevard, #9, Issaquah
Mini Michelangelo (18 months +)

Kelsey Creek Community Park (page 114, 127)
13204 SE 8th Place, Bellevue   (425)455-7688
Clay Expressions (2½–6 years)

Laurelhurst Community Center (page 56–57)
4554 NE 41st Street, Laurelhurst   (206)684-7529, page
Toddler Art (2–3 years)

North Kirkland Community Center (page 116–117)
12421 NE 103rd Avenue, Kirkland   (425)828-1105
Parent/Child Art (2–3 years)

Northwest Center (page 118)   (425)462-6046
9825 NE 24th Street, Bellevue
Pee Wee Picasso (1½–2½ years)

Ravenna-Eckstein Community Center (page 62–63)
6535 Ravenna Avenue NE, Ravenna   (206)684-7534
Ooey Gooey Play (2–3 years)

Renton Community Center (page 119–120)   (425)235-2560
1715 Maple Valley Highway, Renton
Messy Time for 2's (2 years)

Quick Reference Guide

Drop-Off Classes

Ballard Community Center (page 48–49)   (206)684–4093
6020 NW 28th Avenue, Ballard
ABC/123 (2 years)

Bitter Lake Community Center (page 50–51)
13035 N Linden Avenue, Bitter Lake   (206)684–7524
Discovery Corner Juniors (2–3½ years)

Laurelhurst Community Center (page 56–57)   (206)684–7529
4554 NE 41st Street, Laurelhurst
Toddler Art Play Group (2–3 years)

Loyal Heights Community Center (page 58–59)
2101 NW 77th Street, Loyal Heights   (206)684–4052
Infant and Toddler Program Co-op (infant–36 months)

Ravenna-Eckstein Community Center (page 62–63)
6535 NE Ravenna Avenue, Ravenna   (206)684–7534
Tiny Tots (2–3 years)

Dance Classes

All That Dance (page 47–48)   (206)524–8944
5507 NE 35th Avenue, Laurelhurst
Parent/toddler Creative Movement (2–3 years)

Cameo Dance (page 52)   (206)528–8183
7220 NE Weldon Avenue, Green Lake
Parent/toddler (2–3 years)

Quick Reference Guide

Creative Dance Center (page 52–53) (206)363-7281
12577 N Densmore Avenue, Haller Lake
Parent/toddler (1½–3 years)

Dance Fremont (page 53) (206)633-0812
900 N 34th Street, Fremont
Parent/toddler (2–3 years)

Spectrum Dance Theater (page 95) (206)325-4161
800 Lake Washington Boulevard, Madrona
Movement with your toddler (walking–3 years)

Mom with Baby Fitness Classes

Ballard Community Center (page 48–49) (206)684-4093
6020 NW 28th Avenue, Ballard
Morning Step It Up Aerobics

Ballard Family Center (page 49) (206)706-9645
5449 NW Ballard Avenue, Ballard
Moms on the Move

Ballard Olympic Athletic Club (page 50) (206)789-5010
5301 Leary Avenue NW, Ballard
Moms and More Aerobics

Green Lake Community Center (page 55–56) (206)684-4961
7201 E Green Lake Drive, Green Lake
Morning Joggers/Aerobics Babysitting

Holistic Yoga Center (page 16) (206)547-9882
4649 N Sunnyside Avenue, Green Lake
Post-partum Yoga

Quick Reference Guide

Seattle Gymnastics Academy (page 64–65) (206)362-7447
12535 NE 26th Avenue, Lake City
Mommy and Me Fitness

Swedish Medical Center (page 19–20) (206)386-2502
1120 Cherry Street, 1st floor aerobics room
Moms and Babies Exercise

Swedish Medical Center/Ballard (page 20)
(206)789-3857; (206)781-6344
5300 NW Tallman Avenue, Room ABC

University Family YMCA (page 68) (206)524-8613
5003 NE 12th Avenue, University District
Aerobics for Moms

Indoor Playgrounds, Open Gyms & Playrooms

Ballard Community Center (page 48–49) (206)684-4093
6020 NW 28th Avenue, Ballard
Toddler Playroom and Gym Tot Time

Ballard Family Center (page 49) (206)706-9645
5449 NW Ballard Avenue, Ballard

Bitter Lake Family Center (page 51–52) (206)368-0172
13035 N Linden Avenue, Bitter Lake

Bitter Lake Community Center (page 51–52) (206)368-0172
13035 N Linden Avenue, Bitter Lake

Bitter Lake Family Center (page 51–52) (206)368-0172
13035 N Linden Avenue, Bitter Lake

Quick Reference Guide

Crossroads Community Center (page 110) (425)452-4874
1600 NE 10th Street, Bellevue
Playgroup

Delridge Community Center (page 92) (206)684-7423
4501 SW Delridge Way, West Seattle
Toddler Mini Gym

First Steps (page 110-111) (425)392-2095
317 NW Gilman Boulevard, #9, Issaquah
Free community play time

Green Lake Community Center (page 55-56) (206)684-4961
7201 E Green Lake Drive, Green Lake
Toddler Play Center

Highland Community Center (page 112) (425)452-7686
14224 Bel-Red Road, Bellevue
Open gym Toddler Time

Issaquah Community Center (page 112-113) (425)837-3300
301 S Rainier Boulevard, Issaquah
Toddler Time

Magnolia Community Center (page 35-36) (206)386-4235
2550 W 34th Avenue, Magnolia
Tot Gym

Meadowbrook Community Center (page 59-60)
10515 NE 35th Avenue, Lake City (206)684-7522
Preschool Open Gym

Meadowbrook Family Center (page 60) (206)366-9256
10517 NE 35th Avenue, Lake City
Playroom

Quick Reference Guide

North Kirkland Community Center (page 116–117)
12421 NE 103rd Avenue, Kirkland   (425)828-1105
Indoor Playground

Rainier Family Support Center (page 94)   (206)723-8590
Rainier Community Center, 4600 S 38th Avenue, South Seattle
Playroom

Ravenna-Eckstein Community Center (page 62–63)
6535 NE Ravenna Avenue, Ravenna   (206)684-7534
Indoor Playspace, Toddler Open Gym

Renton Community Center (page 119–120)   (425)235-2560
1715 Maple Valley Highway, Renton
Terrific Tots Playground

Shoreline Center Gym (page 66)   (206)546-5041
185th Street and 1st Avenue, Shoreline
Indoor Playground

Shoreline Family Support Center (page 66)   (425)235-2560
17018 NE 15th Avenue, Shoreline
Playground Indoor Playground

Southwest Family Center (page 94–95)   (206)937-7680
4555 SW Delridge Way, West Seattle
Playroom

West Hills Family Enrichment Center (page 122)
12704 76th Avenue South, Skyway   (206)772-2050
Playroom

Index

A
access 9
Alderwood Mall 149–150
Alki Beach 102
Alki Playground 102
All for Kids Books and Music 28, 157
All That Dance 47–48, 182
Anderson Park 132
Anderson Park/Redmond Parks and Recreation 108–109, 178, 179, 181
Ardmore Park 123
Arena Sports 91–92

B
Bagel Oasis 163, 172
Ballard Community Center 48–49, 182, 183, 184
Ballard Community Center Playground 83
Ballard Family Center 49, 177, 180, 183, 184
Ballard Olympic Athletic Club 31, 50, 183
Ballard Pool 29
Barlee's Family Pizza and Pasta 166
Barnes and Noble 28
Bay Pavilion Carousel 32–33
Bayview Park 44

Bellevue Aquatics Center 29
Bellevue Community College 24
Bellevue Family YMCA 31, 109–110
Bellevue Square 150–151
Bells, The 164
Billy McHale's Restaurant 169
Bitter Lake Community Center 50–51, 182, 184
Bitter Lake Family Center 51–52, 177, 184
Bitter Lake Park 73, 176
bookstores 27–28
Borders Books 28
Bovee Park 123–124
Brighton Playground 98
Brown Bag Café 173
Bryant Park 79–80
Burke-Gilman Place Park 80
Burke-Gilman Trail 80–81

C
Cameo Dance 52, 182
Camp Long 103
Carkeek Park 83–84
changing tables 10
Children's Museum 33–34
Circo Circo 173
City of Bellevue Downtown Park 124

classes 9
Clyde Beach Park 124–125
Coleman Pool 30
cooperative preschools 23–24
Cowen Park 69
Coyote Creek Pizza Company 169
Creative Dance Center 52–53, 183
Crestwood Park 132–133
Crossroads Community Center 110, 185
Crossroads Mall 151
Crossroads Park 125
Cucina! Cucina! Italian Café 159

D
Dahl Playground 74
Dance Fremont 53, 183
Dearborn Park 98
Delridge Community Center 92, 184
Delridge Park 103–104
Desert Fire 170
Discovery Park 44

E
East Queen Anne Park 42
Egg Cetera's Blue Star Café 164
Evans Pool 30
Everest Park 133
Evergreen Community Health Care 15–16

F
Factoria Square 152
Family Works 54–55, 177
Farrell-Mcwhirter Park 134–135
features 10
fees 9
First Steps 1111, 175, 181, 185
Fishin' Place, The 170

5 Spot Café 161
food and drink 10
Forbes Creek Park 134
Forest Hill Park 125–126
Frankie's Pizza 171
Fred Meyer 148

G
Garfield Community Center Park 39
Garfield Family Center 39, 177
Gas Works Park 69–70
Gene Coulon Memorial Beach Park 142, 176
Gilman Park 84
Gilman Village 152–153
Golden Gardens Park 84
Grass Lawn Park 134–135
Green Lake Community Center 55–56, 183, 185
Green Lake Park 70–71, 176
grocery store playrooms 147–148
Guild 45th Street Theater/ Crying Room 56
Gymboree 24–25, 175, 178

H
Helene Madison Pool 30
Hiawatha Playground 104
Highland Community Center 112, 185
Highland Park 105
Highpoint Park 105
Hillaire Park 126
Holistic Yoga Center 16, 183
Houghton Beach Park 135
hours 9

I
I-90 "Lid" Park 96
Idylwood Park 135–136
information blocks 9
Iron Horse Restaurant 162

Island Crest Park 96
Issaquah Community Center
    112–113, 175, 178, 185
Issaquah Train Depot Museum
    113–114
Issaquah's Julius Boehm
    Pool 30
Ivanhoe Park 126
Ivar's Acres of Clams 162

J
Jay Berry's 171
Jitters 172
Jonathan Hartman Park 136
Juanita Bay Park 136–137
Julia's in Wallingford 165

K
Kelsey Creek Community Park
    114, 127, 181
Kid Swim 31
Killarney Glen Park 127–128
Kindermusik Beginnings 25,
    180
Kiwanis Park 142–143

L
La Leche League 17
Lake Boren Park 144
Lake City Park 74
Lake Forest Park Towne Centre
    153
Lake Hills Park 128, 176
Lake Sammamish State Park
    143
Lake Washington Technical
    College 23
Lakemont Community Park
    128–129
Lakemont Highlands Park 129
Lakewood Park 106
Laurelhurst Community Center
    56–57, 181, 182
Laurelhurst Playground 79

Lawton Park 45
Liberty Park 144–145
Lichton Springs Park 75
Lincoln Park 106, 176
Little Gym, The 57–58, 92–93,
    114–115, 175, 178
Loyal Heights Community
    Center 58–59, 175, 182
Loyal Heights Playground 88
Luna Park Café 167–168
Luther Burbank Park 97

M
Madison Park 39–40
Madrona Park 99
Magnolia Community Center
    35–36, 179, 180, 185
Magnolia Park 45
Magnuson Park 81
Maple Leaf Park 75
Marymoor Park 137, 177
Matthews Beach 76
Mayfair Park 42
McGraw Street Bakery Café
    161
Meadow Park 138
Meadowbrook Community
    Center 59–60, 185
Meadowbrook Family Center
    60, 177, 185
Meadowbrook Pool 30
Medgar Evers Pool 30
Medina Park 130
Memorial Park 143–144
Mercer Island Boys and Girls
    Club 93–94
Meridian Park 71
Metro Cinemas/Crying Room
    61
Meydenbauer Beach Park
    129–130
Mom's Group 115–116
Mothers and Others 116
Mounger Pool 30

Mount Baker Park 99–100

N
Newcastle Beach 145
Newport Hills Park 130
North Acres Park 76
North City Parent
 Cooperative 24
North Kirkland Community
 Center 116–117, 176, 179,
 180, 181, 186
North Kirkland Park 138, 177
North Seattle Community
 College 24
North Seattle Family Support
 Center 62, 178
Northgate Mall 153–154
Northgate Theater/Crying Room
 61
Northwest Center 118, 179,
 180, 181
nursing 10

O
Othello Playground 100
Overlake Hospital Medical
 Center 18

P
Pacific Science Center 36, 176
Paramount Park 90
Pegasus Pizza and Pasta 168
PEPS; see Program for Early
 Parent Support
Pescatore Fish Café 166
Peter Kirk Park 139
Peter Kirk Pool 30
Phinney Neighborhood Preschool
 Cooperative 24
play equipment 10
Playspace at Crossroads Mall
 119, 176
Point Grill, The 168

Pritchard Beach 100
Program for Early Parent
 Support 14, 18–19
public libraries 26–27

Q
QFC 148
Queen Anne Aquatic Center 30

R
Rainier Beach Pool 30
Rainier Community Center
 Playground 101
Rainier Family Support Center
 94, 177, 186
ratings 9
Ravenna Park 71–72
Ravenna-Eckstein Community
 Center 62–63, 180, 181, 182,
 186
Red Robin Restaurants
 159–160
Redmond City Pool 31
Redmond Towne Center
 154–155
REI Downtown Store 37
Renton Community Center
 119–120, 176, 179, 180, 181,
 186
restaurants 158–173
restrooms 10
Richmond Beach 77
Riverview Playfield 107
Roanoke Park 40
Roasted Pepper, The 163
Robinswood Community Park
 131, 177
Rogers Park 43
Ross Park 85

S
Sacajawea Playground 77
Safe 'N Sound Swimming 31
Salmon Bay Park 88

Samena Swim and Recreation Club 120–121
Sandel Playground 89
Santa Fe Café 167
Seacrest Park 107
Secret Garden, The 29, 65
Seattle Aquarium 37–38
Seattle Central Community College 24
Seattle Gymnastics Academy 64–65, 179, 184
Seward Park 101
shade 10
shopping 147–157
shopping malls 148–157
Shoreline Center Gym 66, 186
Shoreline Cooperative Preschool 24
Shoreline Family Support Center 66, 186
South Seattle Community College 24
Southcenter Mall 155
Southwest Family Center 94–95, 176, 178, 186
Southwest Pool 31
Spectrum Dance Theater 95, 183
Spiritbrook Park 139
star rating system 9
Stars 28
Swedish Medical Center 19–20, 184
swimming pools 29–31

T
Third Place Books 29
Thomas Teasdale Park 146
Top Ten Toys 67
Tune Tales 67–68, 180
Twin Ponds Park 90

U
University Bookstore 28
University Family YMCA 68, 179, 184
University Village 156–157

V
Van Aalst Park 140
Victory Heights Playground 78
View Ridge Park 82
Village Theatre 122
Volunteer Park 40–41, 177

W
wading pools 10
Wallingford Center/North 45th Street 157
Wallingford Park 72
Washington Park Arboretum 41
Waterbabies Aquatic Program 31
Waverly Beach Park 140
Webster Park 85
weekend/evening hours 9–10
West Hills Family Enrichment Center 122, 186
West Magnolia Playground 46
West Queen Anne Park 43
Wilburton Hill Park 131
Willows Creek Park 141
Woodland Park Playground 86, 177
Woodland Park Zoo 86–87, 177
World Wrapps 160–161

Z
Zoka Coffee Roaster and Tea Company 165

About the Author

Julia Rader Detering was inspired by her son to write *Bringing Out Baby*. After giving up corporate life to stay at home with her new baby, she soon became restless. So together mother and baby embarked on a quest to find places to take babies in Seattle. After uncovering a wealth of activities and places, they decided to share their findings with mothers, fathers, grandparents and others caring for babies and toddlers. She now continues to use her findings with her second baby boy.

Julia enjoys hiking, mountain biking and exploring the Northwest and beyond. When not out and about with babies and toddlers, she is a freelance writer and stay-at-home mom. She lives in Seattle's Green Lake area with her husband and two boys.

If you have questions or comments regarding this book, please e-mail: bringingoutbaby@hotmail.com.